THE

ASTHMA

BREAKTHROUGH

Second Edition

HENRY OSIECKI

B.Sc. (Hons.), Graduate Dip. Nutr. & Dietetics

VITAL HEALTH PUBLISHING

Health ~ Nutrition

Bloomingdale, IL

GENERAL DISCLAIMER

The information presented in this book is for general informational purposes only and is not a substitute for professional medical advice. Please do not use the information in this book for diagnosing or treating a medical or health condition. You should carefully read all product packaging. If you suspect that you have a medical problem, promptly contact your professional healthcare provider.

Statements and information regarding dietary supplements in this book have not been evaluated or approved by the Food and Drug Administration. Please consult your healthcare provider before beginning any course of supplementation or treatment.

Published by Vital Health Publishing
P. O. Box 544
Bloomingdale, IL 60108
(630) 876-0426 Phone/Fax

Cover inset: Microphotograph of vitamin C crystals with 60 second breath interval pattern by Prof. Spike Walker, UK. Reproduced with permission.

ISBN: 1-890612-22-7

This book is dedicated to

My wife Vera,
and children
Henry, Mariangela and Michael

CONTENTS

INTRODUCTION

One afternoon about two years ago I stopped at the corner shop to buy some milk. My little girl, toddling close behind, immediately spotted the brightly colored packs of snack-foods and decided that she simply had to have some.

A battle ensued as usual, and I explained to the lady behind the counter that my daughter suffered from severe food allergies and asthma. The bright yellow 'cheese' snacks, which she refused to release from her grip, were just the sort of thing to start her coughing. I was well aware of many of the things that caused adverse reactions, but we were far from having her illness under control. It all seemed so frighteningly complex.

The shop assistant then gave me some advice, which proved to be of enormous benefit to our family. She told me how all three of her children were severe chronic asthmatics. Years of intensive medical treatment and constant worry had left their family physically and financially drained.

Their search for an answer to this never-ending problem led them to Henry Osiecki. Finally, after years of ill health, the girls began to get well. Within a short time they no longer needed the drugs which they had depended upon to avoid a life-threatening attack. Some changes to their diet and a nutrient supplement program were all that was needed to bring about this remarkable improvement.

This is just one of countless similar success stories which I have heard about since. Our family is eternally grateful to Henry and his wonderful team of professionals for helping us with many different problems.

I know there is a great need for this book, and that it will help a great many people. Here's to better health and an end to asthma!

— Juliann Bidmead

Treatment of severe asthma attacks must be treated promptly by your doctor. The suggestions given in this book are preventive practices that may reduce the frequency and severity of asthma.

CHAPTER 1

UNDERSTANDING ASTHMA

During the past decade the incidence of asthma in the developed world has shown an alarming increase, with up to 20% of the population affected. The good news is—we now know much more about asthma and its causes, and there is no doubt that most people can learn to **help themselves** to overcome this troublesome condition. With the correct nutritional and preventive measures—asthma **can** be beaten.

One in every ten Americans has asthma. One in eight American children are affected on average, and for many of these, nebulizers and drugs such as bronchodilators are a familiar part of life well before their third birthday. Every year millions of dollars are spent on asthma medication and treatment, not to mention the misery endured by more than 15 million asthma sufferers in the U.S. alone (Journal of Allergy and Clinical Immunology, Dec. 2000). An enormous amount of this expense and suffering could be eliminated if more people understood the condition and were able to approach the causes rather than just attempting to alleviate the symptoms.

Asthma can pose a threat to life, but only to a small percentage of the population affected. Doctors often blame poor patient compliance with drug therapy for many of the deaths that have occurred. Some say that many patients are apathetic about using medication properly, particularly the type that needs to be taken on a regular basis. The problem seems to be largely a lack of information and awareness as well as the patient's failure to realize when an attack has gotten 'out of control'. There is often poor patient-doctor communication and many people are frightened of using prescribed drugs. Obviously the emphasis on patient educa-

1

tion needs to be shifted to the area of prevention and encouragement of self-help to bring about improvement in general health through correct nutrition and lifestyle.

When treating asthma it is not enough to simply dampen or suppress the symptoms as they arise, while ignoring the underlying problem. In fact this can be quite dangerous. Yet, this is exactly what a great many asthma sufferers do when they pay little attention to their general health and simply reach for the 'puffer' when things get a little tight. It is **essential** to ask the question—"What has actually caused the asthma to develop in the first place and what exactly is asthma?"

Asthma is the **result** of a complex bio-chemical process within the body. It is a common misconception that this problem begins and ends within the lungs alone. The health of the body in general, and in particular the immune system, needs to be looked at as the first step in understanding the real nature of asthma.

SYMPTOMS

Most people are well aware of the basic symptoms—a wheeze and/or cough accompanied by varying degrees of breathing difficulty. Asthmatics often complain of a tight sensation in their chest, which can be so severe that they feel they are 'bursting' with air. This can happen when air becomes trapped within the airways making it difficult for the lungs to 'deflate' properly.

Sometimes, particularly in very young children, there is no audible wheeze, just a nagging but often exhausting cough. Some children will cough so much that it causes them to vomit.

Mothers who have never heard their child wheeze, may be surprised when the physician detects wheeze with a stethoscope. It is important to note that a wheeze does not have to be loud to be a problem.

Fatigue is another common problem for chronic asthmatics. Airway obstruction causes a decrease in lung function and extra effort is required to breathe. Fatigue is also caused by a decrease in arterial oxygen levels which is due to the depressed respiration. Carbon dioxide may also be retained as a result of the inability to exhale properly. As well as this, the quantity and quality of sleep may be affected as symptoms occur commonly at night.

DIAGNOSIS OF ASTHMA

As well as noting the characteristic symptoms, a physician may detect abnormalities within the lungs such as congestion or broncho-constriction. Reduced lung capacity can be determined with a simple device known as a spirometer, but because asthma symptoms can come and go, there may not be any obvious signs at the time of consultation with the doctor, particularly with children or those with infrequent attacks. A chest x-ray is sometimes done to rule out other possible causes of the symptoms. A device known as a peak-flow meter can also be used at home to measure breathing capacity. The reading on the meter—known as the peak expiratory flow rate (PEFR)—drops when asthma symptoms are first developing, (often well before they become troublesome) so it is possible for the patient to self-monitor his condition in this way.

Asthma symptoms are reversible—and the patient may feel fine between attacks. However, certain commonly recognized triggers often become apparent, such as exercise or exposure to cold air and other irritants, which makes diagnosis and treatment easier.

Sometimes, particularly in children, 'post-nasal drip' or catarrh may cause a chronic cough, and parents may worry that the cough is due to asthma. This happens when nasal secretions—usually caused by allergy or irritation—run into the throat rather than out of the nose. This is most common in young children who can't blow their nose properly, and like asthma, it is often troublesome at night. Asthma medications will not help this condition, but many of the asthma prevention measures discussed in this book will. Treatment of post-nasal drip may be as simple as reducing exposure to irritants such as pollen and dust and building up health with a good nutritional program.

CHARACTERISTICS OF ASTHMA

The word *asthma* is of Greek origin and means 'panting'. The disease is commonly referred to as 'a reversible airways obstruction', or 'respiratory allergy', although neither of these terms accurately describe the whole problem. Within the overly sensitive lungs of an asthma sufferer certain distinguishing characteristics are seen:

- The smooth muscle wall of the airway becomes swollen and inflamed. This causes the airway to narrow, reducing airflow. Even in people with very mild asthma, examination of the airway with a bronchoscope reveals this reddened, swollen appearance of the smooth muscle. A biopsy (sample) of this inflamed tissue would reveal damage to the epithelium (surface cells) and varying amounts of inflamed cells. These cells consist mainly of eosinophils and lymphocytes—these are types of white blood cells that are activated by the body in the presence of allergy or infection as part of the normal immune reaction. In asthma, the eosinophils can have a negative action causing damage to the airway lining.

- The mucous membrane of the airway produces an excessive amount of mucous. This mucous combines with plasma (a component of blood) which comes from leaky blood vessels in the inflamed airway wall. This causes the mucous to become very thick and sticky, forming a plug in the airway that further restricts airflow. The mucous may also be affected by other factors such as dehydration (fluid loss) of the body.

- Certain cells in the airway lining known as mast cells interact with **allergens** (substances which cause allergic reaction) and release **mediators** such as **histamine**. Most people who have suffered from hayfever symptoms (blocked, runny nose; sneezing; red, itching eyes etc.) have at some time taken an anti-histamine preparation, and so, have some idea of what histamine is. It is one of the main culprits in allergic reaction and causes (in asthma) swelling and constriction of airways, excess mucous production, plasma leak from blood vessels and the activation of inflammatory cells. It is not, however, the most active mediator in this particular condition and antihistamines will not control the symptoms of asthma. Another mediator is **bradykinin** which also causes constriction of airways by contracting the smooth muscle. Perhaps the most important mediator though, is **Platelet Activating Factor** (PAF). This is the greatest cause of blood vessel porosity, and it also causes excessive mucous secretion, constriction of airways and activation of inflammatory cells, especially **eosinophils**. It has been proven to cause **long-term** hypersensitivity of airways. The effects of PAF can take up to three days to fully develop, but they can last for three weeks. PAF attracts eosinophils and then activates them to make more PAF. This process then continues to work in a cycle. It is now believed that PAF, and therefore eosinophils, are the major contributing factors to epithelium damage and airway inflammation. Because of this, asthma has been referred to by some experts as 'eosinophilic bronchitis'. (Nature has provided us with ways of counteracting each of these processes and substances—this will be discussed in detail in Chapter 4).

♦ Nitric Oxide is another inflammatory mediator that is released during an asthma attack. Quenching the activity of this mediator can forestall the cellular damage that may occur during an asthma attack.

THE IMPORTANCE OF THE EPITHELIUM

The epithelium is a **protective barrier** made up of a layer of tightly joined cells in the lining of the airway. Its function is basically the same as the outer layers of our skin—it protects the underlying tissue from invasion by irritating or infective substances.

The epithelial cells also release a natural bronchodilator substance, which assists in keeping the airways open, so obviously, the condition of the epithelium is of great importance to an asthma sufferer. In every biopsy performed on an asthmatic's airways, there has been large numbers of damaged epithelial cells found, and in the mucous there are often large clumps of these cells.

Once the lung (epithelial) barrier is broken down, the airway walls are highly vulnerable. The body's own immune system, the eosinophils literally tear off the lung (epithelial) cells from the lining and these now damaged cells can release the chemicals which will activate the process of chronic inflammation. One reaction then leads to another, each one contributing to the severity of symptoms.

Another effect brought about by the breaking down of the epithelium is the exposure of sensory nerve endings. These nerve endings become inflamed and then release neurotransmitters, which mimic the symptoms of asthma, contributing to a worsening of the overall condition. The mediator, bradykinin also stimulates these nerve endings and it is this substance which is most responsible for inflammatory pain.

In chronic asthma the damage to the epithelium can lead to a layer of fibrosis (scarring) beneath it. This sub-epithelium fibrosis may lead to adhesion of membranes, structural changes and damage to the airways. The fibrosis may come about as a result of long-term, inadequately treated inflammation, so it is essential to control this. It is possible that structural damage of the airways could ultimately lead to very serious conditions such as emphysema and bronchiectasis.

From this analysis of asthma, several important features have become apparent, the most significant being that asthma is much more than smooth muscle contraction of the airway. This contraction has always been considered the major abnormality in asthma, but it is now understood that the prominent feature in asthma is the inflammation. **Asthma is inflammation** of the airways within the lungs and the symptoms of asthma are brought about as a result of this inflammation.

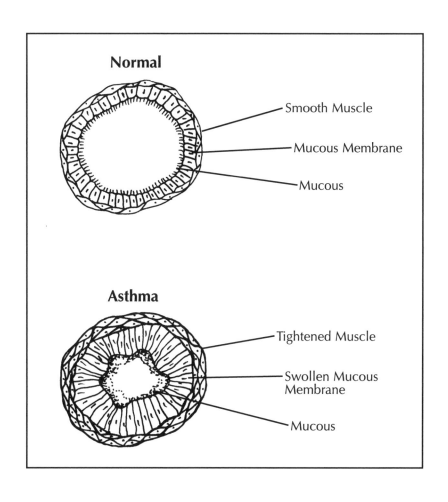

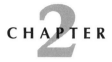

THE CAUSES OF ASTHMA
Who is Affected and Why?

Asthma may affect anyone at any age, but symptoms do seem to be more prevalent in certain age groups. Very young children with asthma tend to have quite frequent symptoms, due to the immaturity of their immune systems and lungs, but often their asthma improves and sometimes disappears completely as they grow older. By adolescence many children are virtually symptom-free, although the asthma can at times return later in life.

A common situation is for a **tendency** toward asthma to persist, even after regular attacks seem to have stopped. Less frequently, a person can have severe, chronic asthma right throughout life, but this situation may well have come about as a result of neglecting the illness early on. **There is no doubt that if asthma is ignored it will continue to recur and worsen**.

Sometimes, asthma may strike for the first time in adulthood (adult-onset asthma) and this type is often the most severe and most frequently fatal, particularly if it occurs after the age of forty.

Even though many of the same things will trigger an attack in both children and adults, there are differences in the asthma process between the two groups. Adults and teenagers seem to be more likely to suffer a sudden, life-threatening attack than small children. Over the years adults have been exposed to greater levels of dangerous irritants (such as cigarette smoke, chemical fumes etc.) and they may develop a very high sensitivity to some of these. The health of young children is usually monitored very closely by parents and doctors, whereas adults tend to take their own health for granted, too often ignoring signs and symptoms until they become very sick. This leads to a further increase in sensitivity and inflammation, which may cause more damage.

Children tend to improve and 'build up' quickly once the asthma triggers are removed and their immunity is boosted, making them more resistant to further reactions. Adults, however, may not be able to strengthen their resistance so easily if a lot of damage has been done.

A woman who was treated recently for chronic asthma was doing extremely well after some adjustments to her diet and lifestyle. After one night at a party where she was exposed to large amounts of cigarette smoke, she suffered a severe asthma attack, and it took several months for her to fully recover. This is one example of how severe sensitivities can develop and wreak havoc on health.

Many people who have asthma are known to be **allergic** to a variety of substances. It is very common to find that an asthma sufferer has a family history of allergy. Hayfever, eczema, chronic sinusitis, allergies to various foods, drugs or chemicals etc. can often be found in different members of the family. Quite often, the asthma sufferer himself will have other allergic conditions, most commonly chronic sinusitis and hayfever. Children with asthma very often seem to have eczema to some degree, and doctors often note that the two conditions seem to go 'hand in hand'. This has been found to be related to the release of **leukotrienes**—inflammatory mediators that seem to affect both the skin and the lungs. Allergic individuals (and often their families) are referred to as 'atopic' (on the surface) in medical language.

THE IMMUNE SYSTEM

Throughout life the body is exposed to a huge amount of microscopic, yet potentially lethal, invaders (such as bacteria or viruses). Almost everything that we eat, drink, breath or touch contains these tiny organisms, many of them extremely harmful. Without some kind of protection, the body simply could not cope with this constant attack from the world around it, and people would be dying from things as simple as the common cold.

Our protection is known as the immune system and it consists of special cells within the body, which are able to recognize and fight invaders. The immune system must be functioning properly in order to defeat these natural enemies. It is normal for people to have a certain amount of colds and flu, etc., but if our immune systems are healthy we should be able to 'shake them off' without too much trouble. If our immunity is not up to scratch, we tend to 'pick things up' much more often, become much sicker and take longer to recover.

However, our immune system needs to be trained to respond to bacterial and viral infections appropriately. It is well known that if animals are exposed to a sterile environment their longevity is reduced quite dramatically. The immune system needs to be exposed to parasites (worms), bacteria and viruses; otherwise it becomes unbalanced. Recent evidence suggests that the increased incidence of allergic reactions in the developed world is due to the excessive cleanliness of our livable environment. In the undeveloped world where many children are exposed to a variety of parasites and infections, allergy rates are relatively low.

The biochemical difference between the allergic and non-allergic individuals is the relatively large amounts of an immune mediator called interleukin-10 being released by the non-allergic individual. This mediator has anti-inflammatory properties and is released by the immune cells when exposed to parasites and the like. It is interesting to note that the lung macrophage (immune cells) of asthmatic patients is deficient in producing interleukin-10. So in an individual whose immune system has not been primed properly, an unbalanced response to allergens, viruses and bacteria occurs. The individual becomes more sensitive to allergens and reacts inappropriately.

ALLERGY

When certain potentially harmful substances enter the body, the immune system reacts by producing antibodies against them. An example of this occurs when vaccines (antigens) are given to produce resistance to a particular disease such as measles. It is possible to determine a person's immunity (resistance) to many diseases with a blood test that can detect the presence of antibodies to that particular disease.

When an allergy occurs, the body mistakenly targets substances that are not normally harmful, and produces a certain type of antibody (IgE antibodies) to them. These antibodies bind to mast cells in the body, and the mast cells then release mediators such as histamine when the allergen enters the body. Once these antibodies are present, the body is sensitive to the substance, and further exposure to it will bring about an allergic reaction. Allergy is therefore an **inappropriate response** by the immune system, and the immune system could be said to be **over-reactive**. (The word 'allergy' is of Greek origin and means 'altered reaction'.)

Some people are sensitive to such an extensive range of things that their lives are affected dramatically, but usually it is not too difficult to live with allergy if good health is maintained and allergens are identified and avoided. Much can be done to reduce the harmful effects of allergens with nutritional treatment.

Allergy may be responsible for a number of health problems, ranging from migraine to skin rashes to gastrointestinal symptoms. It would seem that not only asthma but also allergy in general is becoming more prevalent. An allergy or intolerance of some kind seems to be the rule rather than the exception with people in the modern world. Environmental pollution, chemicalization, food refining and additives place new demands on the body's system. It is really no wonder our body's natural chemistry is 'out of whack' and we are developing all of these ailments.

ALLERGY... OR INTOLERANCE?

There is often confusion about whether an adverse reaction to a food or other substance is caused by allergy or intolerance. There is a difference between the two terms—true allergy always involves an immunological response, whereas intolerance generally does not. For example, people who are lactose intolerant, (lactose is the sugar in milk) are not allergic to milk. The reason they become sick when they drink milk is because they are deficient in the enzyme need-ed to digest the lactose in the milk. The term intolerance generally implies an abnormal adverse reaction that has not been proven to involve an immune mechanism. Allergy and intolerance can and often do exist together.

The causes of asthma are complex and are not always allergy related. Chemical imbalances in the body which are brought about by disease, drugs, diet, etc. may cause some-one to be susceptible to asthma—all that is needed then is the 'trigger' to actually bring about an attack. Hormonal imbalances such as thyroid disease, premenstrual tension or adrenal exhaustion may precipitate the onset of asthma. A bout of pneumonia, pesticide exposure, heart disease, antibiotics or vaccines may cause damage to the lungs lead-ing to a predisposition to asthma.

ALLERGY TESTS

There are several medical methods of testing for allergy, but unfortunately they are often inaccurate and limited in the information they can provide. Skin tests involve placing a drop of an extract (such as a food or pollen) on the skin (usually of the inner forearm) and then lightly scratching through the drop. Some tests are also done by injecting extract just beneath the surface of the skin. An allergic reac-tion is noted if a reddened lump appears. These tests cannot be relied upon as the only means of allergen identification, as it is possible to be highly allergic to a substance and yet have a negative skin test result.

Sublingual testing is performed by placing a drop of an extract under the tongue—directly behind the lower front teeth. The substance is rapidly and efficiently absorbed into the bloodstream from this site.

Positive (allergic) test results are recorded within 2–5 minutes of ingestion. This technique is also used to deter-mine a 'neutralizing' dose of a phenolic substance or of the allergen itself that is then used to control allergy symptoms.

RAST (radioallergosorbent test) and cytotoxic tests involve a blood test, and again the results are often inconsistent.

IgE levels

Raised serum immunoglobin E (IgE) is usually indicative of food allergy. However when testing for cow's milk allergy, intestinal mucosal IgE plasma cell levels is more sensitive than serum IgE or RAST test to cow's milk protein. Double-blind placebo-controlled food challenge (DBPCFC) is regarded as the "gold standard" for diagnosis of food allergens. The food to be tested in this oral challenge is based upon a significant history of reaction to the food and/or RAST or skin test. The food challenge in administered in the fasted state. The challenged dose of food likely to provoke symptoms is approximately 500 mg of lyophilized (freeze-dried) food. This dose is then doubled every 15-60 minutes, depending on the type of reaction that is anticipated. If the patient can tolerate more than 10 gms. of the lyophilized food blended in capsule or liquid without reaction, he is regarded as not clinically reactive. If the blinded portion of the challenge is negative, an open feeding under observation must be undertaken to rule out uncommon false negative challenge.

Keeping a diary of symptoms as well as foods eaten and exposure to possible allergens can provide a great deal of information about what might be causing allergies. Carefully planned elimination diets are a very useful way of determining food allergy (Refer to Chapter 7)

Chemical Sensitivity or the allergic tendency of an individual can be inherited. However, allergic tendency, with no previous family history of allergy, can also be acquired in a number of ways. Hypersensitivity may follow viral infections such as mononucleosis or viral pneumonia, or severe emotional reactions such as grief. The most common incitement appears to be low-grade, long-term chemical exposure, although a short-term high-level exposure, such as seen in industrial accidents, may produce similar effects.

There is apparently no consistent pathway by which the immune system mediates chemical hypersensitivity or loses its control mechanism and begins to sensitize inappropriately to chemicals. The pathways used by the immune system to develop this phenomenon not only

SUBSTANCES OR CONDITIONS THAT MAY PRECIPITATE FOOD REACTIONS

1. ADDITIVES AND CONTAMINANTS

Dyes	Tartrazine

Flavoring and Preservatives
- Nitrates and nitrites
- Monosodium glutamate and glutamate (free glutamate is present in mushrooms, tomatoes, and peas)
- Sulphating agents, metabisulphite
- Sodium benzoate

Toxins
- Bacterial (Botulism, staphylococcal intoxication)
- Mushroom toxin
- Mycotoxins (alflatoxin)
- Sea food associated — Saxitoxin (shell fish)
  - Scombroid poisoning
  - Ciquatera poisoning (mainly from reef fish snapper)
  - Infectious organisms
- Parasites (giardiasis, trishinosis)
- Viruses (hepatitis)
- Insect parts
- Mould antigens

Accidental contaminant
- Heavy metals (Lead, copper, cadmium, mercury)
- Pesticides
- Antibiotics

2. GASTRO-INTESTINAL DISEASES

Structural abnormalities
- Hiatus Hernia
- Internal obstruction

Enzyme deficiencies
- Lactase deficiency
- Pancreatic insufficiency
- Cystic fibrosis
- Other diseases mentioned in the introduction

3. ENDOGENOUS PHARMACOLOGIC AGENTS
Caffeine, Theobromine, alcohol
Histamine
Tryptamine, Tyramine, Dopamine, Phenylethlyamine, Serotonin, i.e. Vaso-active amines

4. OTHER
True allergic reactions
Coeliac disease
Hormonal problems

vary from chemical to chemical but from exposure to exposure, and certainly differ from individual to individual.

There are also the secondary effects or pathways of allergic inflammation. For instance, gastrointestinal symptoms range from vague indigestion to full-blown colitis (inflammation of the colon). These may result in nutritional deficiencies.

The deficiencies begin with increasing sensitivity of the immune system to food. Generalized inflammation of the gastrointestinal tract due to food sensitivity often causes poor nutrient absorption that leads to vitamin and mineral deficiency. Eventually the individual may become deficient in digestive enzymes, which in itself will initiate food intolerance or sensitivity. With increasing vitamin and mineral deficiency and enzyme deficiencies, the end result is an inability to detoxify chemicals, giving rise to more food and chemical sensitivities. **Thus a vicious cycle is set in motion that will only be overcome by judicious supplementation of vitamins, minerals and digestive enzymes.**

Common Chemical Exposures that Cause Chemical Sensitivity

1. **Terpenes**—These are natural, volatile chemicals released from plants. They normally give the characteristic odor or scent of the plant, e.g., odor of fresh pine needles, orange, eucalyptus, cloves, jasmine. The level of terpene exposure depends on the time of year, the highest concentration is present during the warmest part of the year.

2. **Hydrocarbon fuels**—Natural gas, petrol fumes, coal gas, and kerosene. Gas stoves or ranges can be a source of gas leakage in homes. Parking station attendants and petrol attendants are in the high-risk group for this type of sensitivity.

3. **Synthetic ripening of fruits,** such as bananas may liberate potentially harmful residue of the ripening gas ethylene. Commercial coffee that is gas roasted is another example.

4. **Formaldehyde products** are notorious for their adverse reactions in sensitized individuals. Hidden sources of

formaldehyde exposure are plastics, chipboard, home insulating material (foam type), nylon carpets, mouth washes, wood veneer, latex paints, detergents, soaps, hair setting solutions and shampoos. Wash all clothing and towels before using as these may be preserved with formaldehyde or other chemicals.

5. **Perfumes**, heavily scented cosmetics, deodorants, sprays, tobacco, scented soaps, nail polish, strong cleaning solvents and synthetic clothing or garments have all been implicated in chemical sensitivity. Beauticians and hairdressers should be aware that some of their symptoms such as headaches, irritability and fatigue may be due to these scented products.

6. **Pesticides**, herbicides and agricultural chemicals must also be considered as potential problems in some individuals.

7. **Artificial colorings** and flavorings.

8. **Chlorinated water** is also a common culprit.

9. **Synthetic Clothing** may create skin irritation and restrict perspiration.

Symptoms of chemical sensitivity vary quite widely and include headache, irritability, fatigue, asthma, hyper—or overactivity, restlessness, anxiety, sluggish thinking, malaise, muscle pain, arthritis, etc.

NOCTURNAL (NIGHT TIME) ASTHMA

Many people who suffer from asthma have at least once been woken in the middle of the night by an attack. Parents frequently notice that their child's symptoms seem to appear or worsen within hours of being tucked into bed. There may be a trigger such as a drop in ambient or body temperature, but the major contributing factors to night-time asthma symptoms are hormones.

While we are asleep our levels of adrenalin and cortisol naturally drop. Both of these hormones are involved in maintaining normal dilation of the airways and control of tissue swelling. (Adrenalin is often given by injection as an emergency treatment for severe asthma and allergic reaction as it causes rapid reduction of airway swelling.) Both of these hormones also inhibit the release of inflammatory mediators, including PAF, which cause asthma symptoms. During sleep there is also a slight fall in lung function which is completely normal and quite insignificant—if you don't have asthma. To an asthmatic, however, it places yet more strain on the already troubled airways.

Snoring can also causes trouble for people with asthma, as this causes a disruption in the normal breathing pattern. A weak soft palate—a common factor in snoring, particularly in older people, can often be strengthened with physiotherapy, or nasal administration of continuous partial airway pressure (CPAP) can be of value in nocturnal asthma.

Another possible contributing factor to nocturnal asthma is oesophageal reflux or hyperacidity. Although this can cause irritation of the airways at any time, it is often worse at night when lying down, particularly if food has been eaten recently before going to bed. Elevating the head of the bed (by at least 6 inches) can be helpful. See also guidelines for good digestion.

Circadian rhythms can play a role in nocturnal worsening of asthma. Peak lung function occurs at approximately 4 p.m. and the lowest level (of lung function) at around 4 a.m. Over 90% of night asthma occurs between 10 p.m. and 7 a.m. Circadian changes in lung function ranging from 10–50% in asthmatics compared to 5–8% in normal individuals can occur in patients suffering from asthma.

Possible explanations for this increased variation are as follows:

- Bronchial responsiveness to inhaled triggers is increased during night hours

- Levels of eosinophils, neutrophils (white blood cells), superoxide and histamine increase in the airways in the early morning hours.

- Cholinergic or vagal (i.e. nerves) tone increases at night.

- The number and physiological functions of beta 2 adeno receptors (receptors that cause bronchodialation) are significantly reduced from 4 p.m. to 4 a.m.

Chronic sinusitis/rhinitis and/or post nasal drip are frequent problems in nocturnal asthma patients. Treatment of this problem can reduce the frequency/severity of nocturnal asthma.

COMMON TRIGGERS OF ASTHMA
Viral infections

Colds and flu are common precipitating factors.

Candida albicans

This is a fungal organism that is most commonly known as 'thrush'. It is normally present in the intestine in small quantities, but it has the ability to multiply and migrate to other areas where it can cause a variety of problems. This can happen when immunity is poor and also when antibiotics are taken. Oral contraceptives and anti-inflammatory drugs can also cause an overgrowth. As a cause of asthma, candida can infect the mucous lining of the airways and stimulate PAF. (See Chapter 1) Some other symptoms of candida infection are fatigue, headaches, and irritability, joint pain and irritable bowel among others. There are several other types of fungus that may also cause problems.

Pollens

A wide range of grasses and plants contain pollens that become airborne and are then inhaled. They are a common cause of allergy and asthma but what most people don't realize is that they can cause problems even if you are not allergic to them. Pollens are highly irritating to mucous membranes in the nose, throat and lungs, and although they may not be truly allergic to them, some people are more sensitive to them than others. Exposure to diesel fumes is known to sensitize the delicate lining of the nasal passages causing a more severe reaction to pollens in those individuals.

Dust and dust mites

A great many people have found relief from allergy and asthma by taking steps to remove or at least reduce dust from their environment. Like pollens, dust mites are extremely irritating even to non-allergic individuals and it seems they are a very common cause of upper-respiratory problems. The introduction of cold water washing has increased the exposure to dust mites in clothing and bedding. It requires a temperature of 70 degrees centigrade (hot water washing) to destroy these dust mites in clothing. Higher exposure to these dust mites means greater frequency of asthma attacks in sensitive individuals.

Mold

If mold is a problem, symptoms are usually found to be worse in humid, damp, musty conditions. Mold becomes airborne very easily and many people are sensitive to it.

Metabisulphites

Metabisulphites and various other preservatives are used on some foods to retain their color and fresh appearance. Studies have shown these additives to be responsible for 66% of childhood asthma. (See Chapter 4)

Salicylates and Phenols

These are chemicals that occur naturally in some foods and are very similar to aspirin. (The chemical name for aspirin is acetylsalicylic acid.) It is believed that 21% of childhood asthma is related to salicylate sensitivity. (See Chapter 4)

Food additives

Many people, especially children, are known to be sensitive to various artificial colors, flavors and preservatives. Tartrazine), a yellow color which is found in a wide range of foods, seems to be particularly troublesome. This is especially true in someone who is sensitive to salicylate or aspirin.

Artificial colors and other additives may also cause defects to certain enzymes which are known to be deficient in food-intolerant people and which are needed to detoxify certain food compounds. Monosodium glutamate (MSG) is a 'flavor enhancer' which is known to cause severe reactions in some people.

There are many important reasons for avoiding artificial food additives as much as possible, especially if asthma or any other health problem exists.

Cigarette smoke

Cigarettes contain up to 2000 toxic substances including pesticides, arsenic, ammonia and cyanide... say no more.

Chemical fumes and air pollutants

Fumes from household and industrial substances such as paint, cleaners, glues, etc. can often be a serious problem. One particularly dangerous pollutant is sulfur dioxide gas that is thought to have caused an extremely high incidence of asthma in areas near power stations that emitted the gas as fallout. Even very strong odors may disturb the breathing pattern so as to trigger an attack. Long-term, low-grade exposure may be just as hazardous as short-term, high-level exposure, and sensitivities may develop to a number of other substances as well. There has been a definite link found between chemical sensitivity and food intolerance. As the body is required to break down an increasing load of toxins and chemicals in our food, water and air, our detoxifying enzymes can become damaged or even destroyed causing sensitivities and illness.

Animals

Fur and dust from cats, dogs and other animals can trigger allergic reactions and asthma in some children and adults.

Exercise

Exercise can trigger an attack in some people, especially if they exert themselves suddenly or for a prolonged period of time. Other activities that alter the breathing pattern such as laughter or panic attacks are also capable of causing asthma symptoms.

Cold air — Variation in ambient and body temperature

Exposure to cold air, particularly if it is dry, can precipitate an attack. A drop in body temperature and also very cold food or drinks may well cause problems.

Aspirin

Approximately one third of asthmatics react adversely to aspirin. For headache relief, use the headache relief spray on the forehead (providing the person is not reactive to it) or a calcium-magnesium supplement.

Food

The foods most commonly associated with asthma are as follows: cow's milk (29%), egg (7%), chocolate (5%), soy formula (5%), corn (4%), rice, citrus fruit and apple (2% in each case). A wide range of foods and food chemicals may cause adverse reactions and this is discussed in detail in Chapter 4.

Indigestion

Esophageal reflux can irritate airways and trigger asthma. Esophageal reflux may be due to hypochlorhydria, i.e. lack of stomach acidity. The food, instead of being digested, ferments, increasing gas pressure in the stomach.

Drugs

Certain medicines, especially aspirin, drugs containing salicylates and the non-steroid anti-inflammatory drugs, can contribute to or cause a severe asthma attack in sensitive individuals. Sulphonamide antibiotics such as Septrin may also pose some risk. Beta-adrenergic blocking agents such as Inderal should not be taken by anyone prone to bronchospasm.

(See Chapter 3 — Drug Dangers)

Emotional Stress or Trauma, Adrenal Exhaustion

Anxiety, emotional outbursts, grief, fatigue, etc. can precipitate or contribute to asthma symptoms.

Chronic Sinusitis /Allergic Rhinitis

Postnasal drip can initiate an asthma attack.

Other

Almost anything that causes narrowing or obstruction of the bronchial tree may be associated with wheezy and asthma-like conditions. For example: foreign matter, pneumonia, heart disease, insecticide exposure, including fly sprays; tooth paste, fluoridated water, house-hold chemicals, detergents, polyester clothing, paints, carpets, hair sprays, air conditioning, nickel exposure, cholinergic (cholesterol-reducing) drugs or any substance that releases PAF within lung tissue.

Summary

There are two main factors contributing to the increased rate of asthma in the developed world. They are:

(a) **The priming of the immune system towards more inflammatory reactions due to:**

1. The over-consumption of omega 6 oils (safflower, sunflower oils) that tend to prime the immune system to an inflammatory mode.

2. Relative nutrient deficiency, particularly of vitamin B6, C, magnesium, zinc and omega 3 fatty acids. These nutrients play a significant role in regulating the immune system.

3. The excessive cleanliness of the early childhood environment that results in a poorly trained immune system.

The immune system primed by these factors tends to over-react to any stimuli. So the exposure to chemicals, dust mite, or infection causes an over exaggerated immune response, and if these reactions occur in the respiratory structures or tissues, asthma is usually the result.

(b) The introduction of cold water washing in the domestic household.

This has increased individual exposure to dust mite in clothing and bedding, as a temperature in excess of 70 degrees centigrade is required to destroy them. This increase in allergen stimuli acting upon a primed immune system can result in asthmatic symptoms.

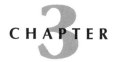

CHAPTER

MEDICAL TREATMENTS
FOR ASTHMA

Drugs are often necessary to treat asthma. Certainly in the case of severe asthma attacks, fast, efficient medical treatment can save lives. However, far too many drugs are misused or relied upon too heavily. Often simple steps could be taken to improve health and prevent asthma without them, or at least with much less of them. Suddenly discontinuing any regular drug is certainly not advised, but it is possible for many people to gradually reach the point where they no longer need pharmaceutical medications.

All drugs have some risk of side effects, and drugs used to treat asthma are certainly no exception.

There has been some recent publicity about the life-threatening potential of certain asthma drugs. The sympathomimetic bronchodilators (drugs that work like adrenaline) such as Ventolin™ and Berotec™ are the focus of this attention. Their use has been linked to heart damage, although this is more likely to occur when they are used frequently over a period of time and without any supporting preventive measures.

Bronchodilators work to open the airways by relaxing smooth muscle spasm—they do not have any effect on the major characteristic of chronic asthma—the inflammation. It is for this reason they have been referred to as a 'band-aid treatment'—they may help to improve breathing for a time but actually do nothing to help the underlying condition. One doctor referred to the use of bronchodilators alone as 'painting over rust'.

Bronchodilators do have an important role to play in alleviating severe asthma symptoms but they should not be the first and only lines of treatment in the long term. The **cause**, and not just the symptoms, must be dealt with.

GENERAL INFORMATION

When a drug is taken, a series of physiochemical events occur within the body. First, the drug typically combines with cell receptors on the cell surface. This is followed by the drug effect, which may be localized (within a limited area), or systemic (affecting different and diverse organ systems in the body). There are many factors, which affect individual absorption, distribution, metabolism and excretion of a drug.

Drugs may be administered orally, where they may react with the contents of the stomach and affect drug absorption. Liquid forms of oral drugs are usually more quickly and completely absorbed. They may be injected intramuscularly (into muscle), subcutaneously (just beneath the surface of the skin), or intravenously, where they are placed directly into the bloodstream and are immediately and more completely utilized. Many drugs used for asthma are inhaled and act directly on the tissues within the lungs. They may also enter the bloodstream via the lungs. Drugs can also be absorbed into the bloodstream in the form of suppositories and skin creams, ointments etc.

The amount of individual body fat, fluid and muscle mass greatly influences the absorption and distribution of drugs. So too does age, nutritional status, underlying illness and the condition of the digestive system. Individuals may also vary greatly in the manner and speed at which they metabolize drugs. In some, metabolism is very fast and larger doses may be required than for others who have a slow rate of metabolism. If metabolism is very slow, a standard dose may have toxic effects.

Elderly people often have decreased liver and kidney function as well as less muscle mass, consequently needing lower doses to avoid toxicity. Young babies also need careful monitoring as their metabolic enzyme systems and kidney function are not fully developed. Anyone with liver or kidney problems needs special care due to the extra risk of drug accumulation, altered effect and toxicity. Some people with highly active liver enzyme systems (rapid acetylators) can develop a rapid build up of toxic metabolites (substances produced when the drug is metabolized) when treated with certain drugs.

ADVERSE REACTIONS

Drugs are prescribed when it is thought that they will be of therapeutic benefit to a patient. However, there is always some risk of side effects occurring with any drug and a decision must be made (usually by the doctor) as to whether the benefit outweighs the potential risk.

Some side effects are very common and predictable, such as the drowsiness caused by antihistamines. Other more severe reactions may require discontinuation of the drug. Some people may be genetically susceptible to certain drug effects and others may be hypersensitive or allergic to a specific chemical or ingredient.

All drugs must be measured carefully and taken strictly as prescribed—and only by the person they have been prescribed for. It is very important to watch for any signs of possible adverse reactions and to report them to the doctor immediately.

DRUGS DURING PREGNANCY AND LACTATION

There are few drugs, which have the 'all clear' for pregnant women. All drugs should be avoided during pregnancy unless absolutely essential to the mother's health, especially during the first trimester when fetal organs are forming and development is most rapid.

Breastfeeding mothers should avoid all drugs unless essential—as most will pass into breast milk. Drug levels are highest shortly after a dose, so it is important to breastfeed just before a dose rather than after. Some drugs must never be taken by pregnant or breastfeeding mothers and all 'over the counter' drugs should be checked with a doctor.

DRUGS AND CHILDREN

Children differ from adults in the way they absorb and metabolize drugs. They take longer to digest stomach contents and the transit time through the small intestine is longer, causing oral drugs to be more completely absorbed. A child can also absorb topical (applied to the skin) drugs more rapidly as the epidermis of their skin is comparatively thinner. It is important to remember that where drugs are concerned, children are not just a scaled-down version of an adult and some drugs prescribed for adults could be very dangerous to a child.

*Some tablets are not meant to be crushed as they are designed for slow release. Check first.

DRUGS USED IN THE TREATMENT OF ASTHMA

BRONCHODILATORS (BRONCHOSPASM RELAXANTS)

These work to open the airways by relaxing muscle spasm—they usually have little or no effect on the inflammatory processes or mucous. Adrenaline (epinephrine) is a bronchodilator and is usually the drug of choice for emergency treatment. In this instance, it is given by injection and works very rapidly to open the airways. However it is also a potent heart stimulant. Common side effects include fear, anxiety, tenseness, tremor, weakness, dizziness, rapid heartbeat and vomiting, even with small amounts. Prolonged administration of this drug can cause severe metabolic acidosis and liver and kidney damage, as well as intolerance to adrenaline, so it is important to get asthma under control and avoid emergency situations. Medihaler Epi™ is adrenaline in an aerosol inhaler, and recommended dosage should never be exceeded.

There are many other bronchodilators, which are known as sympathomimetic amines, and they are all fairly similar in their action and effects. These can be divided into two major groups:

1. Short-acting Beta 2 Agonists that include the following drugs: **Fenoterol, Salbutamol, Terbutaline,** and **Orci-**

prenaline. These drugs stimulate beta 2 adrenergic receptors that are present on airway smooth muscle and thus cause bronchial dilatation. They also effect beta 2 receptors on mast cell and prevent the release of mediators (chemical messengers).

2. Long-acting Beta 2 Agonists that include **Eformoterol**, **Salmeterol**. These drugs stimulate beta 2 receptors on airway smooth muscle resulting in long lasting bronchodilatation, usually in excess of 12 hours.

Side effects associated with beta 2 agonists use include anxiety, tension, nausea, headache, restlessness, insomnia, tremor, excitement, dizziness, rapid heartbeat, lowered blood pressure and flushing. Overuse may cause a serious heartbeat irregularity and a severe fall in blood pressure. Inhaled forms may cause dryness of the mouth and irritation of the throat. Propellants contained in aerosols may also cause problems such as heartbeat irregularity.

There is now evidence that the sympathomimetics may be quite detrimental to health in yet another way. It has long been known that they block the early allergy-bronchospasm reaction but do nothing for the late reaction. This is a serious concern as it means that a patient may feel better after a dose, while in fact his condition is worsening, and he may not gain relief from a later dose once the symptoms flare again. Also, by blocking the early allergic reaction, the normal cough reflex is suppressed (coughing and sneezing are natural ways of expelling irritants). This blocking effect can cause an increase and accumulation of mucous.

The following is a list of some of the common sympathomimetic bronchodilators.

BEROTEC™ (Fenoterol) Aerosol, nebulizer solution, tablets and elixir. Use of this drug has been linked to a number of deaths. Drug literature states that 'fatalities have been reported following excessive use of sympathomimetic amines'. Studies have shown that cardionecrotic effects (death of heart tissue) may occur with high doses and prolonged use.

VENTOLIN™ or **RESPOLIN**™ (Salbutamol) Inhaler, syrup,

injection, nebulizer solution and (Ventolin™ only) rotacaps. This is the most commonly used inhaled bronchodilator. Reports have shown that some people can develop a tolerance to the effects of Salbutamol and it may cease to alleviate symptoms.

BRICANYL™ (Terbutaline) Tablets, elixir, aerosol, nebuhaler, nebulizing solution, injection. This is commonly used in children in the elixir form and most parents whose children have taken Bricanyl™ are well aware of the 'hyping up effect' it induces. This effect is not such a problem if the dose is kept to the absolute minimum and measured with the strictest accuracy, but as with all other sympathomimetics, there are many possible adverse reactions and risks involved with prolonged use.

ALUPENT™ (Orciprenaline) Tablets, syrup, inhaler, injection.

EPHEDRINE™ & FEDRINE™ Tablets.

SERVENT™ (Salmetrol) This is a long acting beta 2 agonist.

IPRATROPIUM™ (Atrovent™—Aerosol, nebulizer solution).

This is an **anticholinergic bronchodilator** and is quite different to the sympathomimetics as it has a fairly localized rather than systemic action and effect. Side effects are reportedly minimal but caution is advised in people prone to urinary retention and constipation. Acute angle closure glaucoma is a possible risk in some people. Atrovent™ is usually recommended for moderate asthma. There are no known adverse effects on the heart with this drug. As with the other bronchodilators, it provides only symptomatic relief and does not help the inflammation or mucous problem.

Other bronchodilators commonly used in asthma treatment are the **theophylline based drugs**, (NUELIN™, THEO-DUR™, ELIXOPHYLLIN™, QUIBRON™, CHOLEDYL™, BRONDECON™). Theophylline is usually given orally as capsules tablets or elixir (it is also available in suppositories and by injection). Some of the tablets are designed for slow release and should not be crushed or chewed. **Theophylline** is a potent cardiac stimulant, diuretic (increases urine flow), as well as a respiratory and central nervous system stimulant. People with high blood pressure, heart problems, or hyperthyroidism need to be very careful if using this drug. Overweight people should receive a dose based on ideal rather than actual body weight.

The most frequent side effects associated with **theophylline** use are: nausea, vomiting, heartburn, abdominal discomfort, headache, rapid heartbeat, insomnia and anxiety. Overdose can cause gastrointestinal bleeding, visual disorders, confusion, vertigo and palpitations. Occasionally, after excessive amounts, sensitive people may develop maniacal behavior, severe vomiting, delirium and convulsions. Theophylline blood levels may increase with a high carbohydrate diet, heart and liver problems, and with the use of antibiotic erythromycin, anti-ulcer drug cimetidine (Tagamet™), antihypertensive drug propranolol (Inderal™) and allopurinol (Zyloprim™) used in the treatment of gout. High blood levels of course, means an increase in the risk of side effects. **Theophylline** interferes with vitamin B6 and B1 metabolism and can give rise to a deficiency of these vitamins. Many leading experts now consider theophylline to be a very poor drug for asthma with unacceptable side effects. However, there is some evidence that theophylline may inhibit the inflammatory process to some degree by blocking the late asthma response. **If a dose of inhaled bronchodilator fails to give the usual relief, medical attention must be sought immediately**.

When taking any of the bronchodilator drugs it is very important to check with a doctor before taking any over-the-counter drugs such as cough medicines or cold tablets as the combination could be dangerous.

Sodium Cromoglycate (Intal—Aerosol™, spincaps, nebulizer solution).

Sodium Cromoglycate is quite unlike any of the other drugs used in asthma management. It works by stabilizing mast cells and preventing the release of certain mediators. **Sodium Cromoglycate** is not a bronchodilator and it does not alleviate the symptoms of an attack. It works as a preventive medication and can be successful when it is used prior to allergen exposure or exercise; however it is not effective in everyone. It is often used on a regular basis. **Sodium Cromoglycate** is considered to be a very safe drug, although it has been implicated in certain immunological changes leading to inflammatory conditions of the heart, lungs and muscles after excessive use. Possible side effects are transient bronchospasm and irritation of the throat and trachea, skin rash, headache, dizziness, nausea and unpleasant taste. The bioflavonoids rutin and quercetin work in a similar way to **Sodium Cromoglycate**.

STEROIDS

These are without question, the cause of most concern for asthma sufferers. The possible side effects are many and often serious, particularly with long-term or improper use. They are used when chronic asthma is severe and not well controlled by other methods. Steroids control and prevent inflammation in a number of conditions as well as asthma and are taken on a regular basis, often in combination with bronchodilators.

The steroids used to treat asthma are known as corticosteroid hormones and they are synthetic replicas of steroids naturally produced by the body. (These are not the same as anabolic steroids, which are used to build muscle—corticosteroids, are catabolic—rather than build up tissue they break it down.) The pituitary and adrenal glands are the centers that control the body's natural production of these steroids. Steroid drugs interfere with production of natural steroids by suppressing their release from the adrenal glands. If this interference continues for long enough natural steroid production can cease completely. This situation is known as adrenal insufficiency and can be extremely dangerous. It is for this reason that REGULAR STEROIDS SHOULD NEVER BE STOPPED SUDDENLY.

Steroids have a major impact on many body functions—they are involved in the metabolism of fat, protein and carbohydrate and also the regulation of fluid and electrolytes. Prolonged therapy can result in cataracts, osteoporosis, change in fat distribution and roundness of the face (moon face), high blood pressure, high blood sugar, retarded growth in children (after as little as six months of regular therapy), thinning of the skin and impaired wound healing, muscle weakness and loss of muscle mass, excessive or abnormal hair growth, decreased resistance to infection, behavior changes, congestive heart failure in susceptible patients, and gastric ulcer, possibly with perforation and bleeding. Even short-term use can result in weight gain, sodium and fluid retention, potassium depletion and decreased resistance to infection. As these drugs can have such profound systemic effects, the smallest possible dose to achieve benefit must be calculated. Some of the corticosteroids used to treat asthma are:

The inhaled corticosteroids—Beclomethasone, Budesonide, Fluticasone.

Other steroids include **Prednisone**, **Prednisolone**, **Dexamethasone** and **Betamethasone**.

Brand Names that contain these steroids are as follows:

Sone™, Deltasone™ (Prednisone), Delta Cortef™, Panafcortelone™ (Prednisolone), Celestone™ (Betamethasone), Dexmethsone™, Decahedron™ (Dexamethasone).

Beclomethasone (Becotide™, Aldecin™) is a relatively new corticosteroid, which is inhaled using a metered aerosol or Rotacaps. It is thought to be much safer than oral forms of steroids. The only adverse reactions reported are dryness of the mouth and throat, and candidiasis of the mouth and throat. Rinsing the mouth and throat after a dose may help to prevent these effects. As with all corticosteroids, Beclomethasone should only be used for short lengths of time and in the smallest therapeutic dose when other methods fail to control asthma.

MUCOLYTICS

These drugs act on the mucous secretions associated with asthma. Mucomyst™ (inhalant) has been developed using **n-acetylcysteine** (a derivative of the naturally occurring amino acid, L-cysteine) to 'break down' the mucous, making it less thick and sticky. There is some danger with this drug as a significant increase in liquefied mucous may occur after use and bronchospasm can worsen. It may cause side effects such as mouth inflammation, nausea and excess nasal mucous, in some individuals.

Bromhexine (Bisolven™) is a similar drug but is available in tablet and elixir form. This initially increases liquidity and volume of mucous but after several days the amount of mucous decreases. Bromhexine may increase the response to bronchodilator drugs, but it may not be effective in the presence of infection. Side effects include: nausea, abdominal discomfort, diarrhea, headache, vertigo, and sweating and skin rash.

DRUG DANGERS FOR ASTHMA SUFFERERS

It is important to remember that aerosol drugs often contain propellants such as fluorocarbons, and that many elixirs contain preservatives, artificial colors and flavors (including tartrazine), and sugar—all potentially hazardous substances. Medications are exempt from labeling laws; therefore, additives are not listed on bottle.

There are some drugs that need to be avoided completely by many people with asthma. **Aspirin** and the non-steroid anti-inflammatory drugs can be particularly dangerous and have caused severe hypersensitivity reactions in sensitive people. It is important to remember that **aspirin** is available under a number of different proprietary names (Bufferin™, Ecotrin™ etc.) and that it is included in a number of preparations including cold tablets. **Aspirin** (acetyl-salicylic acid) and the non-steroid anti-inflammatories all have an effect on prostaglandin's in the body and may aggravate bronchial smooth muscle spasm. Studies suggest that people with asthma would best avoid all of these products even if obvious hypersensitivity reactions have not occurred. Approximately 20% of asthmatics are sensitive to aspirin.

The anti-inflammatories, which should be avoided, include: **Diclofenac, diflunisal, ibuprofen, indomethacin,**

ketoprofen, ketorolac, mefenamic acid, naproxen, phenyl butazone, piroxicam, sulindic, tiaprofenic, tenoxicam, diclofenac sodium+misoprostol.

People prone to asthma attacks should always avoid sedatives as these can severely depress respiration. Antihistamines are quite useless in the treatment of asthma, as histamine is only one of many mediators released in the body during asthma. Unfortunately, many people who are prone to asthma also suffer frequently with other allergic disorders such as hayfever or hives, for which they might take an antihistamine preparation. The problem is that asthmatics do not respond well to most antihistamines. These medicines present considerable risk in two ways. First of all, the cough reflex is suppressed, which may cause an accumulation of mucous in the lungs, and secondly, the drugs have a drying and thickening effect on the mucous. This could lead to the formation of mucous plugs in some cases, and to subsequent lung collapse.

Not all antihistamines affect the lower respiratory tract, but some, which definitely should be avoided, include: **promethazine** (Phenengan™), **cyproheptadine** (Periactin™) and **brompheniramine** (Dimetrap™, Dimetane™).

Sulfonamide preparations that contain **sulfamethoxazole** such as Septrin™, Bactrim™ and Resprim™ can also be dangerous to a few people with asthma.

Another class of drugs known as beta-adrenergic blocking agents which is commonly used to treat angina pectoris, high blood pressure, heart dysrhythmias and migraine should not be used by anyone prone to asthma. These drugs may cause or aggravate bronchospasm and should not be used by anyone with allergic tendencies. They also decrease the effectiveness of asthma treatments. These are the nonselective beta-blockers such as **alprenolol, oxprenolol, sotalol, timolol** and **propranolol**.

Oral contraceptives may produce asthma exacerbation, while long-term use or high dose of postmenopausal hormone replacement therapy increases the risk of asthma.

It is very important, if you have ever had asthma, that a doctor prescribing medication for another disorder is aware of this.

All drugs have side effects — it is important to be aware of these in order to reduce the possible intake if they are a problem. Always consult your doctor and pharmacist if you are taking a number of drugs for various conditions so as to reduce the side effects of drug-drug interaction.

ASTHMA THERAPY DRUGS—Mechanisms of Action

b-adrenergic agents

Cause smooth muscle relaxation and modulate inhibition of mediator release.

Protect against broncho-constriction and micro-vascular leakage

Adverse effects are dose-related

Drugs of choice for asthma attacks

Theophylline

Relaxes bronchial smooth muscle

Decreases micro-vascular leakage, inhibits late response to allergens, inhibits mediator release from mast cells

Used in conjunction with b-adrenergic agents

Used as sustained release to prevent nocturnal asthma

Corticosteroids

Used for maintenance therapy

Inhibit attraction of polymorphonuclear leukocytes to allergic reaction site, block leukotriene synthesis and increase production of b2-receptors

Sodium Cromoglycate

Use as maintenance therapy, particularly in children.

Inhibits mediator release and reduces hyperactivity

Anticholinergic Agents

Block cholinergic pathways that cause airway obstruction

Often used in conjunction with b-adrenergic agents.
Less commonly used

Leukotreine Receptor Antagonists
(Zafirlukast, montelukast, pranilukalut)
  Brochodilators
  Anti-inflammatory
  Block leukotriene receptors

4

NUTRITIONAL TREATMENT AND PREVENTION OF ASTHMA

The treatment of asthma should consist of two basic approaches—removing or reducing causative factors, and strengthening the body's resistance to inflammation and infection. The importance of nutrition should never be underestimated, particularly when asthma or any other illness is present. If exposed to the wrong environment for long enough, the body can reach a point where it becomes more sensitive to negative stressors, causing a need for a great deal more positive nutrition and cleansing.

Our nutritional status forms the foundation of our health and wellbeing. It seems that the old adage 'you are what you eat' is known by everyone—but hardly ever taken seriously. Most people understand and accept the fact that when they don't look after themselves and eat properly they become 'run down'. It is also commonly known that being run down leads to all kinds of health problems and a lowered resistance to illness in general. Unfortunately many people tend to forget this basic wisdom as they rush about in their day-to-day activities.

WHAT IS NUTRITION?

Nutrition is the process by which nutrients are taken into and utilized by the body. Nutrients are substances found in food which are necessary for the growth and function of the body and the overall maintenance of health. The basic nutrients essential to health are vitamins, minerals, amino acids (proteins), essential fatty acids/fats, and carbohydrates. Along with fiber and water, these nutrients need to be consumed daily in relative **balance**.

A person's individual nutritional requirements are influenced by many different factors including age, sex, stress, activity level, genetics and exposure to toxins or drugs. Most people are aware of different needs applying to say, men and women, or children and adults, but they may not be aware of the variety of other factors which determine their personal nutritional needs.

Smoking or exposure to pollution causes the absorption of many toxins into the bloodstream and substantially increases the need for many nutrients. Most drugs, and this includes alcohol, as well as commonly consumed substances such as tea and coffee, can severely deplete the body of essential nutrients, again increasing the body's requirements of these.

How well nourished a person is depends on the quantity, quality and type of food eaten as well as the individual efficiency of digestion and absorption. Certain conditions can occur which affect the stomach's ability to digest and utilize food, for example, insufficient hydrochloric acid. If food is not correctly broken down, the nutrients cannot be properly absorbed, but also, undigested food particles can find their way into the bloodstream leading to a possible allergy or pharmacological reaction to that particular food.

Problems affecting the small intestine such as coeliac disease (gluten sensitivity), may cause a severe malabsorption state resulting in extreme nutritional deficiencies if left untreated. Chronic diarrhea, irritable bowel syndrome, liver and pancreas problems are just some of the conditions which may create poor absorption of nutrients—even if the diet is excellent. Most diets aren't excellent though, and what many people consider to be a 'balanced' diet is quite possibly far from adequate.

Food must also be chewed properly and eaten slowly if the digestive system is to function as it should. For correct nutrition and prevention of allergy or intolerance, good digestion is vital.

The Dangers in Our Diet

Everything that is eaten (particularly by someone with allergies or any illness) needs to be considered for its effect on the body. Foods that provide little nutritional value should be replaced by those that do, and foods that contain artificial additives and contaminants should be avoided. Often it is not so much the foods themselves as the chemicals in them that cause the problems. There is an enormous array of food chemicals, which can affect our health in one way or another, and often it is a certain combination of these which is extremely dangerous.

When certain foods are eliminated from the diet because of allergy or intolerance it is vital to ensure that nutrients normally provided by those foods are derived from another source. Supplements are most certainly required by anyone on a restricted diet; however, if the correct balance of nutrients is taken there is usually no need for very large amounts of any of them. Certain people may have a far greater need for some nutrients, though, and this needs to be accurately assessed by a qualified practitioner in nutrition.

Some of the foods and additives that commonly trigger asthma are discussed below.

Cow's Milk

A great many of the allergies that begin in infancy are related to cow's milk. It is recognized that cow's milk is not the best food for human babies, and many people of all ages are adversely affected by it in one way or another. Over the years our culture has developed a firmly entrenched belief that cow's milk and its products should be a major part of our diet, but this belief is now being challenged. How many cow's milk allergy cases must remain undiagnosed because of this view that cow's milk is of fundamental importance to our health!

Milk can cause an increase in the mucous production of the upper-respiratory tract in many individuals. Many children who have suffered from constantly blocked and runny noses have improved once they stopped drinking milk. Asthma, as well as eczema, rhinitis, sinusitis, catarrh and gastrointestinal problems, has been linked to cow's milk intolerance or allergy in a number of cases. This is not to say that dairy products should be entirely eliminated from everyone's diet, but milk does need to be considered as a possible cause or contributing factor to many health problems.

Infants *under the age of one* should not be exposed to cow's milk. There is association between early cow's milk exposure and diabetes later in life.

Cow's milk is a mixture of more than 20 protein components that can cause possible immunological mediated reactions. Casein, beta-lactoglobulin, alpha bet albumin, bovine serum albumin are the most common components in milk that milk allergy patients react to.

Furthermore, there is a significant cross reactivity between milk proteins in cows, goat, and sheep milk.

Eggs

A common food allergen in children is chicken eggs. The egg yolk has been traditionally considered less allergenic than egg white. The egg white contains ovalbumin, ovomucoid and ovotransferrin, which are the primary allergens, ovomucoid being the major culprit.

Cereals

Many cereal grains can induce allergic reactions. A glycoprotein (i.e. protein bound to sugar molecules, alpha amylase-trypsin inhibitor) which is present in wheat has been implicated in Baker's asthma. Profilins (a family of proteins that controls actin polymerization in eukaryotic cells) are prominent allergens in wheat. These possible protein allergens have a cross reactivity with birch tree pollen, grass pollen and mugwort weed pollen. This cross reactivity shows why allergic patients display a variety of sensitivities to different pollen plant species.

Nuts and Legumes

Peanut sensitivity is reasonably common in children and adults. Unlike allergic reaction to milk and eggs, peanut allergies do not resolve with time. The peanut allergen has been found to be an acidic glycoprotein that is common to the vicilin family of seed storage protein. The vicilin proteins are common to many legumes and other plant species e.g. wheat and cotton.

Salicylates

These substances occur naturally in a great many foods in varying degrees. Chemically they are very similar to aspirin; therefore people who are sensitive to aspirin may need to watch their natural salicylate intake.

As well as triggering asthma in sensitive people, salicylates may cause hives (urticaria), hyperactivity in children, and occasionally ulcerative colitis and nasal polyps.

Salicylate sensitivity or intolerance is usually due to poor liver detoxification pathways i.e. glycine conjugation. Supplementation with glycine, vitamin B1, B5, B12 and C will help the body detoxify salicylates.

Metabisulphites

These days much of our food is geared for mass production and processed to withstand long periods of time from the initial harvesting to when it actually arrives on our table. Unfortunately the use of preserving and refining techniques do little for our health.

Metabisulphites are used as preservatives in a range of foods. These chemicals can be quite dangerous to a person who is sensitive to them. Many severe asthma attacks and anaphylactic reactions (a severe life-threatening allergic reaction) have been attributed to sulphite reactions and possibly a combination of sulphites and MSG (monosodium glutamate).

Many restaurants spray foods, especially salad greens, with sulphite to retain their fresh appearance. Shellfish is also commonly sprayed before it even reaches the restaurant to retain its color. Similarly, meat may be sprayed with sulphite before it is put on display on supermarket shelves so that it will retain its red, freshly cut appearance. In addition to this, wine, cider, and beer often contain considerable amounts.

Other foods which may contain medium to high amounts of metabisulphites include: dried fruit (this is available without sulphites from health food stores and has a darker color), commercial fruit juices, commercially prepared

SALICYLATE CONTENT

	Negligible	Low	Moderate	High	Very High
FRUIT	Pear (peeled), Cavendish banana	Papaya, Golden delicious apple, Pomegranate	Pear (with peel), Loquat, Custard apple, Red delicious apple, Persimmon, Lemon, Fig, Rhubarb, Mango, Tamarillo	Passionfruit, Mulberry, Tangelo, Grapefruit, Avocado, Peach, Mandarin, Granny Smith apple, Nectarine, Watermelon, Lychee, Kiwi fruit, Jonathan apple	Sultana (dried), Prune, Raisin (dried), Currant (dried), Raspberry, Red currant, Grape, Loganberry, Black-currant, young-berry, cherry, Orange, Blueberry, Plum, Pineapple, Boysenberry, Guava, Apricot, Blackberry, Cran-berry, Date, Straw-berry, Rockmelon,
VEGETABLES	Potato (peeled), Lettuce, Celery, Cabbage, Bamboo shoot, turnip, Dried Beans, Dried Peas, red lentils, Brown lentils	Green Bean, Red Cabbage, Brussels sprout, Mung bean sprout, Green pea, Leek, Shallot, Chive, Choko	Broccoli, Sweet Potato, Onion, Parsnip, Mushroom, Carrot, Beetroot, Marrow, Spinach, Cauliflower, Turnip, Pumpkin Asparagus, Sweet corn	Eggplant, Watercress, cucumber, Broad bean, Alfalfa sprout	Tomato products, Gherkin, Endive, Champignon, Radish, Olive, Capsicum, Zucchini, Chicory, Hot Pepper
NUTS	Poppy seed	Cashews	Pistachio, Pinenut, Macadamia, Walnut, Brazil, Pecan, Sesame, Hazelnut, Coconut, Peanut, Sunflower seeds		Almond, Water chestnut

	Negligible	Low	Moderate	High	Very High
SWEETS	White sugar, Maple syrup, Cocoa, Carob	Golden syrup, Caramels	Molasses		Licorice, Peppermints, Honey
HERBS & SPICES		Vanilla, Garlic, Parsley, Saffron, Malt vinegar, Soy Sauce, Tandoori		Cinnamon, Cardamom, Black pepper, Pimiento. Ginger, Allspice, Clove, Nutmeg, Caraway, white vinegar, Bay leaf, White pepper	Cayenne, Aniseed, Sage, Mace, Curry, Paprika, thyme, Dill, Turmeric, Worcester sauce, Vegemite, Marmite, Rosemary, Oregano, Garam masala, Mixed herbs, Cumin, Canella, Tarragon, Mustard, Five spice, Mint
BEVERAGES	**Coffee**–Andronicus instant, Pablo instant, Decaffeinated **Other**–Aktavite, Milo, Ovaltine **Alcohol**–Gin, Whiskey and Vodka	**Coffee**–Harris instant,Bushells instant, Bushells Turkish, Robert Timms instant **Tea**–Chamomile **Cereal Coffee**–Dandelion, Ecco, Bambu	**Coffee**–Harris Mocha, International Roast instant, Nescafe instant **Tea**–Decaffeinated, Fruit, Rosehip **Cereal Coffee**–Reform **Other**–Rosehip syrup, Fruit juice, Coke **Alcohol**–Cider, Beer, Sherry, Brandy	**Tea**–all brands, peppermint **Cereal Coffee**–Nature's Cuppa **Alcohol**–Liqueur, port, wine, rum	

'fresh' fruit salad, dried vegetables, instant potato mixes, cordials, soft drinks, desert toppings, flavoring essences, cheese spreads, cheese pastes, hot chips (commercial), sausages and processed meats, pickles—especially pickled onions, corned beef, tomato sauce, commercial salad dressings and chocolates.

Unfortunately, some products may contain preservatives without this being stated on the pack. Some commercial fruit juices are one example of a product that may be contaminated even though they claim to be additive free. There have been cases of asthma improving after all commercial juices were eliminated.

Yeast Foods

Yeast foods such as bread and cheese should be avoided by those with chronic asthma symptoms. Yeast contains the polysaccharide zymosan, which has been found to be a potent stimulator of platelet activating factor (PAF). PAF is the main inflammatory mediator (chemical messenger between cells) involved in asthma (See chapter 1).

MSG

Monosodium glutamate is the sodium salt of glutamate—a naturally occurring amino acid. It is used to artificially enhance the flavor of foods and is found in a huge range of processed and convenience foods. The term 'Chinese restaurant syndrome' came about as a result of the rather heavy use of MSG in commercial Chinese food. In sensitive individuals, it can provoke an extremely severe asthma attack, but it can also cause a range of other nasty effects such as headache, nausea, vomiting, palpitations, sweating and weakness. MSG toxicity seems most likely to occur in people who are deficient in Vitamin B6. MSG was banned from use in baby food by the National Health and Medical Research Council of Australia as it was found to cause brain damage in young animals. It is still found in a large selection of packet and canned foods. There is widespread documentation of its toxic effects in sensitive individuals. Reactions to MSG are usually quite sudden but may take as long as twelve hours to occur in some cases. There are many foods and additives which may trigger an asthma attack in susceptible individuals, and it is essential to identify these if asthma is to be brought under control. Vitamin B6 supplementation can reduce the severity of reaction to MSG.

NUTRIENTS FOR ASTHMA

VITAMIN B6 (Pyridoxine)

This particular nutrient has been found to be extremely helpful for asthma sufferers, and biochemical research suggests that they may have a far greater need for it than most people due to disturbances in their metabolism. Studies have shown repeatedly that B6 significantly reduces the frequency and severity of symptoms in almost all patients tested. Many people have reported almost immediate improvement after taking this vitamin. Many asthmatics have low red blood cell pyridoxine levels.

B6 is found naturally in brewer's yeast, oatmeal, whole grains, meat and egg yolk. Some of the signs which may indicate a deficiency are irritability, depression, low blood-sugar, tiredness, weakness, dermatitis and other skin problems. Cooking and processing causes considerable loss of this nutrient. The usual supplement dose is 25–100 mg. per day. The contraceptive pill, amphetamines, and chlorpromazine interfere with B6 metabolism.

A deficiency in the mineral zinc can induce B6 deficiency by preventing the conversion of vitamin B6 to its active form, pyridoxal-5-phosphate, so when supplementing with vitamin B6, take zinc with it.

VITAMIN C

Vitamin C has a large number of very important roles and has been found to be of enormous benefit in asthma and allergy related conditions. It is needed by the immune system and is necessary for healing and prevention of infection. It is a potent anti-oxidant and has anti-viral and anti-bacterial properties. As well as being essential to combat and prevent infection and inflammation, it also decreases fluid retention in tissues and assists in detoxifying the body—all very important functions to the asthma sufferer. Vitamin C supplementation of approximately 2 gms. prior to exercise can protect from exercise-induced asthma in approximately 45% of patients.

A large number of people are deficient in this vitamin, mainly because it is not stored by the body and must be replaced daily. Processing and cooking also largely destroys it, and it is depleted in the body by many things such as stress, smoking, pollution exposure and alcohol. Adults should always ensure at least 300 mg. per day is consumed but often much more is required. Low intake of vitamin C and manganese is associated with a five-fold increase in bronchial reactivity to a stimulus.

Good natural sources are rosehips, blackcurrants, citrus fruits, capsicum, cabbage, potatoes and pineapple.

VITAMIN B5 (Pantothenic Acid)

This vitamin is particularly helpful for people with allergies, asthma, infections, stress, fluid retention and low blood sugar. Alcohol, coffee, tea, and stress greatly increase the need for this vitamin, and symptoms that may indicate a deficiency include: irritability, fatigue, poor immunity, fluid retention, sore feet and sleep disturbances. Food sources of B5 include: royal jelly, yeast, whole grains, green vegetables, beans, egg yolk, liver and oranges. A large amount is lost in cooking and processing. Between 20 and 200 mg. should be taken daily. In combination with vitamin B1 and choline, it can help regulate the autonomic nervous system

VITAMIN B3 (Niacin, Niacinimide, NAD)

This vitamin has an inhibitory effect on histamine release from mast cells (white blood cells).

VITAMIN B12 (Cyanocobalamin)

This helps to reduce the effects of toxins and is particularly important if a sensitivity to metabisulphites exists. Smoking, diabetes, alcohol and laxative use are some of the factors increasing demand for B12. Strict vegetarians may risk a deficiency. The best sources are liver, spirulina, meat, milk and eggs. 500 mcg. to 1.2 mg. per day is required.

VITAMIN A (Retinol)

This is important for healthy mucous membranes, resistance to infection, healthy skin and eyes, blood vessels and bone growth. Vitamin A can be of great help to people with asthma, bronchitis, sinusitis, skin problems, stress, gastric ulcers and arthritis among other conditions. A deficiency may mean poor immunity, dry skin and eyes, night blindness and poor sense of taste and smell. The best food sources are animal and fish liver, kidneys, eggs, dark green and orange vegetables (like carrots). Daily intake should be 5000–10000 IU.

VITAMIN E (Alpha-tocopherol)

This nutrient is needed for healing, muscle, nerve and blood maintenance and to stabilize cell membranes. Natural sources include egg yolk, wheatgerm, nuts and vegetable oils. Processing causes considerable losses, particularly from wheat. 100–1000 IU is recommended daily. Asthma of five years duration or more is associated with lower serum vitamin E levels.

A combination of vitamin E and C reduces the effects of atmospheric pollutants and help asthma patients breathe more easily in polluted environments.

ANTIOXIDANTS

Although oxygen is essential to life, it can sometimes produce unwanted effects in the body. Toxic substances produced by oxygen such as peroxide, peroxynitrite and superoxide combine with certain molecules in the body to form 'free radicals'—high-energy chemical substances. It has been found that these free radicals may be largely responsible for inflammatory processes, lowered immunity, cancer cell proliferation, cardiovascular degeneration and accelerating the aging process. Once diseased, tissues are more susceptible to free radical damage. Asthma of longstanding is invariably associated with cellular lipid peroxidation.

Nature has provided an answer to this problem with substances to protect cells against negative oxidative processes —antioxidants.

The main antioxidants are: Vitamins B, A, C, E, lipoic acid, Co-Enzyme Q10, beta carotene, manganese, selenium, zinc, L-cysteine, glutathione and gamma tocopherols.

LIPOIC ACID

Lipoic acid and gamma tocopherol are powerful scavengers of the peroxynitrite free radical. Peroxynitrite is a powerful inflammatory mediator of cell death.

CO-ENZYME Q 10 (Co Q10)

Ubiquinone (CoQ10) improves cellular energy production and also inhibits histamine release. Supplement with 100–200 mg./day.

ZINC

Zinc is an extremely important mineral and a deficiency may contribute to poor immunity, poor healing and growth, skin problems, and psychiatric problems. Some people are unable to absorb or retain zinc in their body due to factors such as high iron intake, low hydrochloric acid, old age and bowel and liver diseases. Zinc is found in oysters, liver, meat, yeast, seeds, green leafy vegetable and wholegrains. Daily supplements should be in the range of 10–100 mg.

MAGNESIUM

Magnesium has some very important functions for the asthma sufferer: regulation of body temperature, protein synthesis and normalizing muscle contraction and nerve excitability. It is also a natural anti-histamine, it decreases brochial hyper-irritability and is a good bronchial muscle relaxant. Diets high in processed foods are often lacking in this nutrient and sugar and fats can often cause it to be less easily absorbed. Signs of a deficiency include: poor appetite, nausea, weakness, tiredness, confusion, poor concentration, muscle cramps, bronchial hyper-activity, wheezing and heart rhythm problems. Best sources are wholegrains; green, leafy vegetables; milk, nuts and soya beans. 300–1000 mg. are recommended daily to relax bronchial muscle and reduce bronchial hyperactivity.

CALCIUM AND VITMIN D

Supplementation with these two nutrients decreases airway obstruction in patients with allergic bronchial asthma within 60 minutes. Vitamin D modulates delayed hyper-sensitivity reactions.

SELENIUM

This mineral is an important anti-oxidant and is needed for utilization of essential fatty acids and regulation of prostaglandin synthesis. Natural sources include garlic, brewers yeast, kelp, milk and eggs. Selenium is usually deficient in asthmatic patients.

MOLYBDENUM

This mineral is needed along with vitamins B5, B12 and C to counteract the toxic effects of metabisulphites, sulphur dioxide, and other chemicals. Food refining and agricultural methods have drastically reduced the amount of molybdenum available in our diet. 100–500 mg. is recommended daily.

ESSENTIAL FATTY ACIDS

The nutritional value of fats is very often underestimated. Essential fatty acids—contained in certain fats—play a major role in many of the biochemical processes which sustain life. They also form an integral part of the cell wall in every cell in the body. They are referred to as "essential" because they are vital to health and the body needs a regular intake.

A deficiency in essential fatty acids (EFAs) or an imbalance in the ratio between Omega 6 oils and omega 3 oils can cause the immune system to react inappropriately to allergens and infection. This imbalance causes an alteration in prostaglandin metabolism. Certain prostaglandins are extremely important as they regulate the activity of immune cells and are necessary to control inflammation and allergies.

It is likely that a large number of people, particularly in western society, are deficient in EFAs as a result of their diet and lifestyle. Cigarette smoke, alcohol, pollution and refined and processed foods indirectly deplete EFA activity or supply and inhibit anti-inflammatory prostaglandin synthesis. A major cause of EFA loss is the hydrogenation of polyunsaturated vegetable oils. Hydrogenation (a process used to convert liquid vegetable oils into solid or semi-solid fats such as in margarine and vegetable shortening) destroys EFAs and changes oils into potentially harmful substances. All food oils should be 'cold-pressed' rather than chemically refined.

EFA deficiency can give rise to a number of disorders including: poor immunity, dry skin and eczema, allergies, asthma, poor healing, impaired growth, cardiovascular abnormalities, headache, PMT, lowered fertility and even cancer. Good dietary sources of EFAs are: cold-pressed sunflower, mustard seed, safflower, linseed and soya oils, oily fish such as salmon, herring and mackerel, (fish oil supplements may be taken) and evening primrose oil. Canola oil, kidney and soya beans, and nuts such as walnuts also contain some EFAs. Ideally, a combination of the above sources should be included in the diet as they provide different types of EFAs.

EFAs can only be correctly metabolized if certain co-factor nutrients are supplied in ample quantity with them. These nutrients are the vitamins A, B6, C, and E, and the minerals zinc, magnesium, copper and selenium. Oils such as evening primrose can be well absorbed by rubbing them into the skin of the inner arm or thigh, particularly in children.

The combination of different EFAs is important if inflammation is to be dampened. In the past 30 years the health authorities have promoted the intake of polyunsaturated fats, particularly soya oil, safflower and sunflower oils. These oils are rich in a fatty acid (linoleic acid) of the omega

6 family. Unfortunately this has resulted in an imbalance in our fatty acids (linolenic) from the omega 3 family to such an extent that the ratio between these two acids is an excess of 20:1 instead of the normal 4:1 ratio. The omega 3 family of oils come from linseed and fishes oils.

As a result of this imbalance, the body reacts adversely to triggers of inflammation i.e. the body overreacts by increasing the inflammation reaction and at the same time decreasing immunity. By having the right mix of oils, the body handles inflammation in a controlled way and increases immunity.

I believe that this change in our fatty acid composition has disturbed the balance in our body giving rise to food allergies, asthma and poor immunity. Correcting this imbalance is essential in bringing back the body to normal reactivity. By supplementing with fish oils, i.e. tuna oil, 3–4 times a week decreases asthma symptoms in 40% of patients.

BIOFLAVONOIDS

The bioflavonoids, rutin and quercetin can be particularly helpful for people with asthma. They significantly reduce tissue swelling and inflammation and quercetin inhibits the harmful effect of the mediator bradykinin on smooth muscle. Quercetin is also a good modulator of inflammatory prostaglandins and leukotrienes. Bioflavonoids are found in the rind and to a lesser extent in the pulp and juice of citrus fruits. The skin of other fruits and vegetables and buckwheat also contain some bioflavonoids. Onions are an excellent source of quercetin.

Supplements are sometimes combined with Vitamin C as they enhance its effects. The supplementary range of the bioflavonoid quercetin is 600-1000 mg. /day.

TAURINE

People with asthma tend to have low serum taurine levels, which increase their sensitivity to aldehydes, hypochlorite, petroleum solvents and alcohol.

Supplementation may be necessary (500-2000 mg.).

GLYCINE

Glycine (supplementary range 2-5 gm.) is an amino acid used by the body to detoxify xenobiotics, e.g. salicylates, aspirin. Glycine metabolism can be impaired in the chemically sensitive individual with vitamin B6 dysfunction.

LYSINE

An amino acid that has been found to have anti-viral activity against the herpes virus.

METHIONINE

Methionine is a sulphur amino acid that the body uses to detoxify many xenobiotics. It supports liver function. Supplementary dose is 300–400 mg./day.

VITAMIN B1 (Thiamin)

Approximately 20% of chemically sensitive individuals are deficient in this vitamin. Supplementation often results in improvement in chemically sensitive individuals.

Excess demand for thiamin (B1) occurs from excessive exposure to formaldehyde, alcohols, glycols, or by overuse of the aldehyde detoxifying mechanism. Thiamin acts as an intermediate carrier of aldehyde groups; without it, aldehydes can accumulate in the body. It must be noted that thiamin is very important in energy production. A relative deficiency will cause tiredness, weakness and anxiety. These symptoms are common in chemically sensitive individuals.

OTHER NUTRITIONAL TREATMENTS

GINKGO BILOBA

Ginkgo biloba is a living 'fossil tree', which has been used for thousands of years by the Chinese to cure conditions of the lungs. It contains ginkgolide B that inhibits platelet -activating factor (see Chapter 1). Ginkgo is a potent anti-inflammatory agent, which has shown excellent results in the treatment of asthma. Ginkgo biloba extracts are also rich in quercetin.

GARLIC

Garlic is a natural antibiotic that is highly effective against harmful bacteria. It also has expectorant and anti-fungal properties and has long been used to treat a wide range of disorders, including inflammation and infections of all kinds. Garlic contains selenium, which is an important antioxidant and EFA co-factor nutrient. Garlic oil (25–35 mg.) should be taken daily.

Herbs such as fenugreek, ma huang, thyme, licorice, grindelia, euphorbia and fennel are all beneficial in the treatment of asthma, excess mucous, bronchial spasm, bronchitis and hayfever.

Ginger has anti-inflammatory properties, and chilies contain a substance known as capsaicin which inhibit certain inflammatory processes which occur in asthma.

N.B.

All supplementary dosages refer to adults. Infants and children require lower dosages. Refer to your physician, herbalist or naturopath for advice.

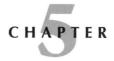

CHAPTER

CHILDREN AND ASTHMA

PREVENTION

Allergies and sensitivities to chemicals such as metabisulfites are major factors in childhood asthma. The predisposition to allergy and other conditions, however, is often developed long before a child is born. Apart from pre-existing hereditary influences, a child's health may be compromised if either parent has poor nutritional status or is exposed to toxins, even before conception. In today's polluted, processed and chemicalized world, there are many factors which can contribute to metabolic and immunological disturbances leading to allergy and illness.

There is a great deal a parent can do to prevent their child from developing these problems. Ensure optimum nutrition, health and fitness (both parents) for at least 6 months prior to conception. Smoking, alcohol and other drugs and chemicals should be avoided. Supplement with a good multivitamin and mineral as well as an essential fatty acid (fish oil or DHA/EPA) supplements to promote optimum nutritional balance. Approximately 20–30% of the female population has elevated homocysteine levels which can adversely affect the development of a child in womb. Supplementing with vitamin B6, folic acid and vitamin B12 is essential in these women to reduce this risk.

During pregnancy, only fresh, natural, unprocessed food should be eaten and all artificial additives and preservatives should be avoided. It is also important to avoid eating very large amounts of one food—small amounts of the widest possible variety should be eaten to prevent the baby from becoming sensitized to a particular food. It is best to limit consumption of those foods that are commonly associated with allergy such as cow's milk and eggs (especially egg whites). No more than one or two eggs should be eaten per week. Pregnant women are often advised to drink plenty of milk to provide calcium, but a baby can become sensitized to the proteins in cow's milk very readily before it is born. Other sources of calcium include almonds (best soaked overnight), legumes, sesame seeds, salmon, tuna, molasses and green leafy vegetables. Calcium supplements are usually prescribed in pregnancy, along with several other nutrients that are needed in greater quantity than usual.

Ensure that nutritional supplements are taken in **balance**. Very large amounts of one could adversely affect the levels and effects of others. Iron, for example, if taken in excess can deplete zinc levels. Zinc is extremely important to the baby's developing immune and respiratory systems, and needs for this mineral are far greater during pregnancy.

Most mothers are well aware of the importance of breast-feeding. Breast milk is the perfect food for a baby, containing a unique blend of nutrients, antibodies, amino acids, enzymes and essential fatty acids that provide optimum protection from allergy and illness. It can cause problems however, if allergens or toxins are transferred from the mother through the milk. Colic, eczema, wheezing and digestive disturbances are some of the conditions which have been known to subside in a baby once the mother stopped drinking cow's milk, for example.

Some women may drink a lot of cow's milk, thinking that it will boost their own milk supply, but the truth is 'you don't need milk to make milk.' While cow's milk may have nutritional benefits, it can and does cause many problems for babies. Recent research suggests that combining supplementary formula feeds with breastfeeding in the first few weeks of life may cause intestinal inflammation and subsequent intolerance or allergy, particularly if there is a family history of allergy. The combination of immune-boosting breast milk and cow's milk foreign proteins should be avoided at this early stage.

A breastfeeding mother whose baby develops skin rashes, upper respiratory mucous, reflux, diarrhea, irritability or sleep disturbances should look carefully at her own diet. Dairy products, eggs, wheat, citrus fruits, chocolate, yeast and peanuts are some of the most common offenders. The breastfeeding mother should avoid all artificial additives and chemicals. Caffeine and aspartame (Nutrasweet™) can cause irritability and gastrointestinal disorders in a baby, and household sprays and insecticides should be strictly avoided. A stringent weight loss diet should never be attempted while breastfeeding as toxins stored in fat tissue can be released into the bloodstream and, therefore, the breast milk. Vital nutrients could also be lost.

It is most important to prevent nutritional deficiencies from developing. Essential fatty acids must not be overlooked, as they are extremely important to the baby's developing immune and neural systems.

With the introduction of solid food come new challenges to the baby's digestive and immune systems. To avoid allergy and intolerance, it is essential not to start solids too early. Each new food should be introduced gradually and only one food at a time should be given while watching for any possible reaction. If an allergic family history exists, it may be wise to avoid introducing common food allergens (such as eggs and wheat) until around twelve months of age. As a general rule, egg white should not be introduced into the diet before 12 months of age—even if there is no family history of allergy.

The first year of a child's life is also critical in terms of chemical exposure. A baby's liver is immature and unable to detoxify many substances, so all artificial additives of any kind should be avoided. Organically grown food is always recommended. Particular attention should be paid to the avoidance of metabisulfites as these are such a common factor in childhood asthma. Ideally, fruit juices and purees should be prepared at home as commercial fruit products may sometimes cause problems, despite preservative-free claims.

Sugar and salt should not be added to meals, and the diet should consist of a variety of fresh, natural unprocessed foods. It would also be worthwhile to limit high salicylate foods in the young child's diet as these are another common factor in the development of asthma in children (See Chapter 4 for information on salicylates and metabisulfites).

The Importance of Digestion

Research as far back as 1931 has shown a strong link between insufficient hydrochloric acid and childhood asthma. When too little digestive acid is present in the stomach, incompletely digested food particles may enter the bloodstream causing an immune reaction and allergy to develop. Studies have shown 80% of asthmatic children tested to be deficient in hydrochloric acid, with the youngest children having the greatest deficiency. Digestive enzymes and hydrochloric acid supplements have been shown to be of significant benefit to many children with asthma (see list of suggested nutritional supplements). Vitamin B12 deficiency is commonly associated with low levels of hydrochloric acid, and this vitamin is particularly important in the prevention of chemical sensitivity.

The Treatment of Childhood Asthma

Asthma in children can almost always be completely overcome with the correct nutritional and environmental control. The following guidelines should be observed.

- ◆ Eliminate sugar, refined and 'junk' food as well as all artificial flavors, colors and preservatives, especially tartrazine, MSG and metabisulfites. Supplements with nutrients that help the body detoxify some of these chemical additives (Refer to chapter 4).
- ◆ Salicylates may be a problem—consider a low-salicylate diet (Refer to Chapter 4).
- ◆ The diet should consist of a wide variety of fresh, natural food (Refer to Chapter 9).
- ◆ Supplements are necessary for the child with asthma (Refer to Nutrients for Asthma, Chapter 4).
- ◆ Learn to recognize which foods or irritants are triggering the child's symptoms. The use of an elimination diet may be necessary.

- It is essential to reduce dust, mold and other irritants as much as possible. Smoking should not be allowed in the home. **Ensure all clothing and bedding is washed in hot water to destroy dust mites** (Follow suggestions in Chapter 6).

- Ensure adequate fluid intake.

- Treat colds, sore throats, ear infections, etc. as soon as they appear with garlic, vitamin C, bioflavonoids, zinc, essential fatty acids and vitamin A. Also avoid milk, refined foods and sugar as these foods increase mucous. Clear congestion with menthol or camphor used with a vaporizer.

- Reduce stresses and tension in the child's environment.

- Encourage the child to breathe through his nose rather than his mouth, especially when air is cold or dry, or when exercising.

- If exercise triggers asthma in the child, it is important that he does not overexert himself. However, **regular, controlled** exercise is essential to increase lung function and fitness. Swimming is a very good exercise for children with asthma and it should be started from an early age. Beware of chlorine in pools as it can be an irritant. The newly popularized salt water swimming pools are preferable as they reduce exposure to chlorine and chloroamines that accumulate in chlorinated pools. Fresh, non-irritant air is important when exercising. A vitamin C supplement can reduce exercise-induced asthma.

- To help improve lung function and to encourage good breathing habits, a child can learn to play a wind instrument such as the flute—or even better, brass instruments like the trumpet, trombone or tuba.

- Encourage good posture from an early age.

- Consider a possible hydrochloric acid deficiency and supplement appropriately (refer to list of suggested nutritional supplements).

- Ensure a regular intake of oily fish or supplement with fish oil.

A child with asthma needs a warm, relaxed, loving environment. It is important that he or she does not feel 'abnormal' or inadequate because he has allergies or asthma and requires special treatment. Every effort should be made to provide interesting alternatives to foods that are disallowed. Children, particularly once they reach school age, can feel they are missing out if their diet and lifestyle is restricted, so maintaining excitement in their life is vital.

If asthma or other illness is chronic and uncontrolled, serious problems can arise affecting both physical and emotional wellbeing.

Repeatedly missing school and social activities can be detrimental to a child's academic and social development. In severe asthma, when drugs must be taken, it is particularly important that a child understands his/her condition and feels positive about himself/herself.

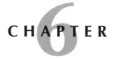

PRACTICAL HELP

CREATING A HEALTHY ENVIRONMENT

There are many simple steps that can be taken to remove or at least reduce the levels of irritants, which trigger asthma. Even if your asthma is only mildly troublesome, it is essential to consider the long-term effect your environment can have on your health. Asthma can and does become worse if it is ignored.

DUST MITE

Dust mites are often found in their largest numbers in and around beds. Careful vacuuming of this area, including the mattress, should be done once or twice a week. Linen should be washed in a 1% tannic acid solution, or hot water (70°C) and dried in the sun at least once a week. The mattress and other surfaces can also be treated with the solution (use a tightly wrung sponge on the mattress and then dry with a hair dryer). The mattress can also be covered with a polythene sheet.

Allow plenty of fresh air and sunlight into the room and be wary of objects in the room that may harbor dust, especially anything stored under the bed. In children's rooms, soft toys are often targets for dust mite populations, so these should be washed and dried in the sun frequently. Bedrooms should be kept tidy and uncluttered and synthetic quilts and pillows should be used (Dacron is ideal). Do not use feather quilts.

The rest of the house should be kept as dust-free as possible by vacuuming frequently and by using a damp cloth for dusting rather than a feather duster. Water chamber vacuum cleaners are a good idea. Fans and air conditioners can be a problem as they circulate dust and other particles in the air.

Carpet is not the ideal floor covering for people with allergies or asthma since it is very difficult to remove all the dust from it. Loose rugs are preferable as they can be washed and put outside to air in the sun. If carpet is very old it is especially likely that it is a major cause of allergy problems as it probably harbors mold as well as dust. Curtains and window areas also need frequent, thorough cleaning. Hardwood floors are preferred over any floor coverings so as to reduce the concentration of dust mites.

MOLD

Microscopic mold spores circulate unseen in the air around us, often wreaking havoc on sensitive noses and airways. Any areas in the home that don't receive adequate ventilation or sunlight should be checked carefully. Pillows, quilts and soft furnishings should be aired in the sun, where possible, on a regular basis. White vinegar can be used to eliminate mold in many areas.

If mold is suspected as a major factor in your asthma, foods containing mold should also be avoided; e.g.

- ◆ foods containing yeast
- ◆ beer, wine and cider
- ◆ buttermilk, sour cream
- ◆ fermented, smoked, pickled foods
- ◆ canned tomato and apple products
- ◆ any canned or preserved food not used immediately
- ◆ refined flour and sugar
- ◆ mushrooms, dried fruit, cheeses
- ◆ food that has been 'sitting' in the fridge for a while

Refrigerators should be cleaned out frequently with vinegar as mold accumulates there quickly, especially around the rubber seals.

Air conditioners and evaporative coolers can harbor mold so these should be checked regularly.

Remember that mold growth is highest in warm, dark, moist conditions.

COCKROACHES

Tiny particles left behind by cockroaches can be inhaled, causing irritation of the airways. These creatures can be dealt with without using highly dangerous sprays and powders. Sealing tiny cracks around the house and cupboards and keeping everything scrupulously clean is the most important step. By not providing them with food or places to hide and breed, you will drastically reduce their numbers. Clean out cupboards in the kitchen and laundry often, especially under sinks, refrigerators and stoves and try some of the natural 'insecticides' or deterrents such as lavender oil. Cockroach traps can be used rather than baits as they do not contain pesticide. A good way of reducing the cockroach population is to spread out a bait mixture consisting of diatomaceous earth, fine borax powder and sugar.

ANIMALS

Animal fur and skin scales are fairly common causes of allergic reaction and asthma, with cats being the worst offenders. It is believed that washing the animal frequently can help, but if a severe sensitivity exists it may be necessary to avoid close contact altogether. Pets should never be allowed in the bedroom, and any inside areas where they are allowed should be vacuumed and cleaned thoroughly.

POLLENS

The plants which cause the most trouble for asthma sufferers are those which rely on the wind for pollination. The larger pollen grains which are carried from plant to plant by insects are not as easily inhaled. On a dry, warm, windy day, thousands of these tiny grains can be circulating in just one cubic meter of air. Areas near busy roads can have very high pollen counts as the currents caused by fast-moving traffic increase their circulation.

The most notorious causes of asthma are ragweed, timothy grass, Kentucky blue grass, Johnson grass, perrenial rye and velvet grass. However, wide ranges of irritant pollens exist, and they vary from one area to another. Ideally, if you have asthma, you should not mow the lawn yourself, but it should be done frequently to prevent the spread of the rapidly growing grass pollen spores that tend to appear almost everywhere. Plants release pollen as they reach maximum growth, so, ideally, they should be attended to before this point. Unfortunately, even if your own garden is 'asthma free,' dry, windy days can carry pollens for miles. So if a severe sensitivity exists, it may be necessary to stay indoors until the wind settles.

Breathing through the mouth, due to nasal blockage or strenuous activity, can cause pollens to be more readily inhaled into the lungs. Diesel fumes should be avoided as these cause the mucous membranes of the nasal passages to become sensitized to pollens.

STOP SMOKING

If you have asthma, it is vital that you don't smoke or allow smoking in your home. When possible, avoid areas where other people smoke as well.

HOUSEHOLD CHEMICALS

There is an extensive range of products designed for domestic use which are bad news for asthma sufferers. Aerosol sprays of all kinds should not be used, and where possible, natural alternatives to potentially harmful chemicals should be found. Some of the most common asthma triggers include oven cleaners, ammonia products, bleach, fabric conditioners, hair sprays and colors, pesticides, air fresheners, perfumes and some cosmetics. Some building materials, glues and paint fumes can cause severe reactions so it is important to avoid these. The home should be kept well ventilated and any room with obvious fumes from glue or paint, etc. should be avoided until the air is clear. It is especially important not to sleep in a room that contains strong odors or fumes. If you have an open fire or wood-burning heater, ensure that it is not faulty as the smoke and dust from these can be a serious problem.

Chlorofluorocarbons (CFC's)—used as refrigerants, aerosol agents and propellants may cause free radical damage to lung tissue.

Toothpaste can induce bronchial spasms, possibly due to artificial flavoring.

OCCUPATIONAL HAZARDS

There are many work environments that may contribute to or trigger asthma symptoms, but it may not be necessary to change jobs if this is the case. You might, however, need to discuss with employers certain aspects such as dust and mold in the workplace, co-workers who smoke, lack of ventilation, air-conditioning which is too cold (a common problem in large offices), etc. Improving your general health and resistance will certainly help, but if your system is under constant stress from irritants and allergens at work, something needs to be done to reduce your exposure.

A wide range of substances can cause occupational asthma. Grain dust and insecticides may trouble farmers and grain handlers. Carpenters and builders may develop asthma after exposure to wood dust, chemicals used to treat wood, glues, paints etc. and hairdressers may react to dyes, bleaches and perming solutions. Careful consideration needs to be given to the types of irritants you may be exposed to for forty hours or so of the week.

An air filter may be helpful, particularly if you live in an area that has a high level of air pollution, or in a farming area where for example, wheat dust or rape seed pollen is a problem. High Efficiency Particulate Air (HEPA) filters have reportedly proved helpful to asthma sufferers. Exercising in polluted air (e.g. jogging by the freeway) is highly likely to produce bronchospasm as the lungs much more readily absorb the harmful substances in the air such as sulphur dioxide. Always exercise in fresh, unpolluted air, and remember to breathe in through your nose rather than your mouth.

TEMPERATURE

The temperature of the house, and in particular the bedroom should be kept at a comfortable level of warmth. In very cold areas it may be necessary to use heating throughout the night as the combination of very cold air and the adrenaline drop which occurs during sleep (see Chapter 2 – Causes of Asthma) may trigger a severe attack. Again, it is important to breathe in through your nose if you are exposed to dry air, as the nasal passages help to warm and moisten the air before it reaches the airways. If you have problems with a blocked nose, it is essential that you do something about this, as healthy mucous membranes in the nasal passages are vital to the person with asthma. (See Chapter 8—Allergic Rhinitis) Air conditioning can be quite hazardous as it dries out the air and is often either too cold or too hot.

It is important not to have the temperature too high, because if you need to go outdoors, the sudden change can lead to bronchospasm. Fan heaters should not be used as these circulate irritant particles and dry out the air too much. In winter the air tends to be very dry anyway, so if you don't own a humidifier, leave some bowls of water around the room which will help to rehydrate the air.

Drinking or eating very cold food can also trigger bronchospasm, whereas hot soups and drinks help to open the airways.

EXERCISE AND ASTHMA

If your asthma is exercise induced, it certainly does not mean that you should give up exercising. In fact, it is more important than ever that you maintain physical fitness – you just need to go about it in the right way:

- Sustained, strenuous exercise causes rapid breathing through the mouth, so that 'unfiltered', dry air is taken in at a faster than normal rate. Endurance sports or activities are not a good idea for this reason. You should choose a type of exercise that enables regular intervals.
- You should not exercise in very cold air. If this is unavoidable, try wearing a mask or scarf over your mouth and nose to help keep the air warm as you breathe.
- Exercise should take place in a non-irritant environment.
- Never exercise without warming up first.
- Swimming is highly recommended as an ideal exercise for people with asthma.
- If you have not exercised for some time, you must start gently and gradually. DON'T overdo it.

- Pre-exercise medication is sometimes necessary, but it must be taken BEFORE beginning if it is to work.
- Supplement with 2 gms. of vitamin C 20 minutes before exercise.
- Consciously breathe through the nose until it becomes a habit.

RELAXATION AND BREATHING

Learning the art of proper relaxation is one of the most important things you should do if you have asthma. A great many people today lead an extremely hectic, stress-filled life, leaving little or no time at all for relaxing. But even those who do take time out may not really know how to 'switch off' or how to get all those knots of tension out of their body.

Chronic tension does terrible things to your physical and mental health, and it drains you of large amounts of vital energy. A person who is under constant stress and strain and who feels tired and depressed is much more likely to develop illness, and much less likely to get better.

Apart from the basic health benefits provided, relaxation takes on an even more important role for the person with asthma. Medical studies have proven that the severity of an asthma attack can be dramatically reduced if the patient is taught to relax and breathe properly when symptoms appear. The feeling of being unable to breathe during an attack is terrifying, but panicking causes a chain reaction of muscle tension which ultimately constricts airways further, making breathing more and more difficult.

It is very important that time is set aside every day to practice breathing and relaxation exercises. Yoga is extremely beneficial, but a simple routine of lying down, consciously relaxing each part of the body and breathing slowly and deeply through the nose for ten minutes or so will help enormously. There are some other suggestions for breathing and relaxation in Chapter 7.

THE PSYCHOLOGICAL ASPECTS OF ASTHMA

Many people have heard the rather dubious term, 'nervous asthma'—they may have even had it applied to them.

Unfortunately, a number of people suffering from asthma have been made to feel emotionally or mentally inadequate because it has been implied that their illness has a psychosomatic basis. Asthma is NOT a disease of the mind, and it is not something that people, especially children, should feel embarrassed about. There is no doubt that asthma can be triggered or aggravated by emotional upset, but there is always an underlying physical problem to begin with.

If stress or emotional upset often triggers your asthma, it would obviously be wise to confront this area, either by relaxation therapy or counseling, for example. It is not only upsetting to think that an illness is 'all in your head', it can be quite dangerous, as the person who thinks this way could seriously neglect the very real physical aspects of their condition. Don't label yourself an 'asthmatic', think of yourself as 'a person who has asthma' (and who is doing something about it!).

NUTRITIONAL TREATMENT

1. Determine which chemical gives the worst reaction. This chemical may, in sufficient dilution, be used in sublingual treatment in controlling reactions.
2. Filter or boil all drinking water.
3. Use toxic cleaning products sparingly.
4. Reduce the use of plastics, toxic paints and varnishes. When painting, use odorless alkali-based paints.
5. Do not wear synthetic undergarments or clothes. Cottons and woolens are usually safe. Do not dry clean clothing and use simple soaps for washing.
6. Do not use kerosene heaters during the winter. Heating should be electrical or solar based.
7. Electric stove in preference to a gas stove or range should be installed. If this is not possible, ensure adequate ventilation within the cooking area.
8. Insulation material and floor coverings should be inert. Rock wool insulation is usually satisfactory. Preferably hard, inert materials such as stone, terrazzo, hardwood,

cement, brick, and terra-cotta tiles should be used for flooring. Be careful of wool carpeting with latex or rubber backing.

9. Soft plastics, such as plastic bags, wrapping, window screens, plastic containers, vinyl seating, plastic table-cloths, and other plastic furnishing should be removed from the home. Use glass containers, cellophane bags, aluminum wrapping and wall-paper.

10. If you are chemically sensitive, remove any synthetic or rubber furnishing in the bedroom. Use all cotton pillows and mattresses instead. Electric blankets should not be used. Cane or hardwood, leather, wool or other natural fiber should be used in furnishings. Cabinets may be made of formica, hardwood or metal but not of chipboard and without silicone chalking.

11. Other sources of chemical exposure are from chemicals released from glued parts and grouting, particularly when heated; chemicals used in hobbies such as photography, photocopying machines; pesticides used indoors or in the garden; timber impregnated with chemicals; tobacco smoke.

12. Avoid all formulated foods or drugs that contain artificial flavorings, coloring or chemicals.

13. Supplementation with vitamins, minerals and amino acids is essential to improve the body's detoxification ability. (Refer to chapter 4)

14. Avoid paracetamol (acetaminophen) for headache relief as it lowers lung glutathione levels and exacer-bates asthma symptoms. Aspirin should also be avoid-ed as it can cause adverse reactions in approximately 20% of asthma patients.

NUTRITIONAL SUPPLEMENT

Supplements suggested below will reduce the inflammation and hopefully improve the metabolism of these chemicals. The nutrients such as taurine, B1, B5, glycine, methionine, B12, and folate need to be taken regularly to improve toler-ances to chemicals.

1. Vitamin C can improve tolerance to many chemicals. However, in a few individuals, it can increase chemical toxicity. In these individuals, alkali or bicarbonate of soda, one hour after meals may be of great benefit

2. Digestive enzymes should be taken with every meal.

3. Hydrozyme or apple cider vinegar, one teaspoon in water with meals, may aid stomach digestion.

4. Fish oils or linseed oil, 1–2 dessert spoons per day, may reduce inflammation.

5. Ginger is a thromboxane synthetase inhibitor and can reduce inflammation.

6. Vitamin B5 and taurine may reduce formaldehyde sensitivity.

7. Vitamins B6 and C may reduce MSG sensitivity.

8. Vitamin B12, glycine and molybdenum supplementation may reduce metabisulphite and sulfite sensitivity.

9. Try a neutralizing dose of quercetin and rutin.

10. Zinc supplementation can be used for tartrazine sensitivity.

11. Alkali may need to be taken in between meals to improve digestion.

12. Avoid all formulated foods or drugs that contain artificial flavorings, coloring or chemicals.

13. Supplementation with vitamins, minerals and amino acids is essential to improve the body's detoxification ability.

NUTRIENT SUPPLEMENTATION OPTIONS

For mild acute attacks of asthma the following should be taken:

Black coffee (no sugar or milk)—contains the drug theophylline—1 cup. This will only work if coffee is not used on a regular basis.

Pyridoxine-5-phosphate	10 mg.
Quercetin	600 mg.
CoEnzyme Q10	100 mg.

Calcium   400 mg.
Vitamin D   100 i.u.

Nutritional Supplement Options

Multi-vitamin capsule should be taken by every asthmatic

Tuna Oil	3 tsps./ day	(Rich in omega 3 fatty acids)
Pyridoxal -5-Phosphate	10 mgs. x 3 per day	(Activated vitamin B6)
Vitamin C as		
Ca & Mg salts of vitamin C	2 gm./day	(Improve immunity)
Zinc (as sulfate	20 mg./day	(Activates Vitamin B6 metabolism/ improves immunity)
Vitamin B12	500–900 mg./day	(Detoxifying nutrient, reduces homocysteine levels)
Folic Acid	400–800 mg./day	(Detoxifying nutrient, reduces homocysteine levels)
Quercetin	600–1000 mg./day	(Anti-inflammatory, antiviral, inhibits PAF)
Alpha Tocopherol		
(Vitamin E)	600 mg./day	(Antioxidant, immune stimulant)
Gamma Tocopherol	50–100 mg.	(Antioxidant, quenches the peroxynitrite ion)
Co Enzyme Q10	90–180 mg./day	(Improves cellular energetics, prevents anaphylactic reactions)
Taurine	1000–2000 mg./day	(Improves chemical detoxification, suppresses bronchial response to PAF)
Magnesium		
(as ascorbate/orotate)	200–400 mg./day	(Broncho-Muscle relaxant, improve cellular function)
Tyrosine	400–1000 mg./day	(Improve adrenal exhaustion, precursor of adrenaline)
Lipoic Acid	50–100 mg./day	(Antioxidant, reduces inflammation)
Pancreatin(Enzyme)	1 Capsule with meal	(Improves digestion)
Ginkgo biloba Extract	160 mg.	(Inhibits PAF)
Ginger Extract	375mg.	(Inhibits thromboxane synthesis, diaphoretic)

N.B. All supplementary dosages refer to adults. Infant and children require lower dosages. Refer to your Physician for advice.

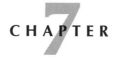

ALTERNATIVE TREATMENTS
FOR ASTHMA

There are quite a variety of approaches to health problems which do not fall within the mainstream of orthodox medicine. Not all of these 'alternatives' will be discussed here, but many of the treatments which have proved helpful to people with asthma and other disorders are well worth consideration. A great many people are enjoying the benefits of the natural therapies, and interest in these areas is continuing to grow at a rapid rate.

HERBALISM

It is a sad fact that when the 'synthetic' age arrived, bringing with it scores of synthetic (and expensive) drugs, grandma's tried and true remedies were largely forgotten. The use of medicinal herbs goes back a long, long way, and enormous amounts of information about herbs and their benefits has been gathered over the centuries.

Some of the main herbs used in the treatment of asthma and lung conditions include: licorice, grindelia, ma huang, euphorbia, mullein, fennel, thyme, marjoram, colt's foot, sage, parsley, and black cohosh. The substances contained in these herbs can work in a number of ways. Some have anti-inflammatory or anti-bacterial properties, others are able to relax smooth muscle and help to clear mucous. Most of the herbs have multiple therapeutic properties. Some of the herbs, such as mullein, can be made into an infusion with boiling water for inhaling. Mullein tea is a good lung strengthener, but must be strained to remove the fine hairs that can otherwise irritate the throat. Many herbs are unsuitable for use during pregnancy—and some should not be used by breast-feeding mothers. It is recommended you seek professional advice to maximize the benefits from this form of medicine.

NATUROPATHY

As the name suggests, naturopathy uses natural therapies to promote good health and to treat and prevent illness. It comprises a commonsense approach to health, emphasizing the body's own healing abilities, treating the whole person and not just the symptoms of an illness. Treatment is directed at a structural, biochemic and emotional level. Naturopathy does not treat disease in the way that medical drugs or treatments do—rather, it provides the body with the support needed to heal itself from within, naturally.

Elimination of toxins, and a healthy, natural diet and lifestyle are the major components of the naturopathic approach. Most importantly, naturopathy encourages a positive attitude and promotes faith in the inner strengths of the body. This alone is powerful medicine.

ACUPUNCTURE

Acupuncture has been used by traditional Chinese physicians for thousands of years. It is now increasing in popularity in the Western world, although it was viewed with considerable skepticism for some time.

Acupuncture is based on the concept of energy pathways, referred to as meridians, which run throughout the body and pass through major organs. The energy or 'life force' which moves along these pathways is known as Chi. Certain key points on the body give direct access to a particular aspects of a meridian, and it is at these points where fine needles are inserted to stimulate the required area.

Chi is said to flow freely and continually throughout the body in a balanced way when a person is healthy. Illness occurs when the Chi is disturbed or obstructed. Acupuncture is said to normalize these interruptions in the energy flow, thereby alleviating symptoms. Tied in with the concept of Chi are the balancing forces of Yin and Yang. Yin and Yang are considered as opposites—when in balance, the body is healthy.

CHIROPRACTIC

Chiropractic is quite widely accepted and used, although not always fully understood. Most people think of chiropractors as people who treat back pain, but the concepts involved are far more complex.

The basic idea of chiropractic is that manipulation of the spinal column can normalize energy flow to internal organs by relieving pressure on nerves in and around the spine. By clearing obstruction of nervous energy flow, proper elimination of toxins (via the lungs, kidney, and bowel) can occur.

Chiropractic treatment encourages basic principles of good health including posture, exercise, correct breathing and nutrition. The dorsal vertebrae (mid-section of spine) are involved in disorders of the lungs, hayfever, catarrh and inflammation as well as several other conditions.

OSTEOPATHY

Osteopathy is a manipulative therapy similar to chiropractic in its basic principles. It is concerned primarily with the structure and correct alignment of the musculo-skeletal system which in turn affects the nervous system and general functioning of the entire body. Many conditions including asthma have been known to improve with osteopathic therapy. People who suffer from asthma often develop muscle rigidity of the upper back, chest and shoulders which only makes their condition worse and can lead to chronic pain from muscle spasm as well as pressure on nerves. Osteopathy can correct this type of problem.

'It is necessary to know the spine and what its natural purposes are, for such knowledge will be requisite for many diseases.'—Hippocrates

HOMEOPATHY

Homeopathy involves the use of very small amounts of medicines which in larger doses could mimic the symptoms of the disease being treated—the basic idea being that 'like cures like'.

This method is said to activate the body's inner energies and natural healing ability leading to a more complete and safe cure. Homeopathic practitioners believe in treating the whole body and not just the symptoms. Homeopathy is very well recognized in Britain where there are a large number of established homeopath.c hospitals and clinics. The royal family has apparently used the services of homeopaths for generations. A wide range of disorders have reportedly been treated with great success by homeopathic methods.

Some of the homeopathic remedies used in the treatment of asthma include: aconite, arsenicum album, ipecachuana and kali carbonicum.

HYPNOTHERAPY

Many people with asthma have apparently responded well to this form of treatment. When in a state of hypnosis or trance, a patient is said to be 'receptive' of suggestions put forward by the therapist. These suggestions are aimed at removal of symptoms via the subconscious mind. No one can deny the power of positive thinking, and hypnotherapy utilizes this concept. Stress and anxiety can worsen or even trigger asthma in many people, so if hypnotherapy or any other method relieves that anxiety it may have an important role to play. Many people have learned through hypnotherapy to remain calm when they feel an attack approaching, and this has helped to reduce the severity of symptoms.

ALEXANDER TECHNIQUE

This is a method aimed at re-educating the muscular system to achieve physical and mental wellbeing. The Alexander technique involves becoming aware of incorrect movements or positions of the body and relearning the correct ones. Many people place unnecessary strain or tension on certain muscles and this can become a habit—this method can help people to break these habits which may be causing them physical harm or mental anguish.

For the person with asthma, it may be helpful to become aware of muscles that might be misused as a result of chronic wheezing and coughing. Correct posture and breathing are also of utmost importance to the asthma sufferer, and these can also be taught with this technique.

YOGA

The deep relaxation which can be gained through practicing yoga can be immensely helpful to people with asthma. Improved awareness of the body, and deep, efficient breathing are some of the important benefits which yoga can provide. Yoga, as it is practiced today in the West, consists of a series of special postures combined with deep breathing and often with meditation to enhance physical and mental wellbeing. The yoga postures or 'asanas', combined with abdominal breathing, improve all respiratory functions, increase lung capacity and develop strong muscles and elastic tissues. Pranayama (breathing exercises) teach breath control and keep airways clear. Blood circulation is improved and proper elimination of waste is enhanced. Yoga can revitalize the body and regulate the flow of 'prana'—the life force.

A study carried out at the Yoga Biomedical Trust in Cambridge, showed 88% of the 226 people with asthma and bronchitis received positive benefit by practicing yoga.

NEGATIVE ION THERAPY

This form of therapy is based on the concept that ions (electrically charged molecules) in the air around us can significantly affect our health and wellbeing.

Various researchers over the years have concluded that negatively charged ions are beneficial, whereas positive ions can be harmful. Positive ions predominate in polluted areas and also in rooms where there is electronic equipment. They also rise sharply just before a thunderstorm. Levels of negative ions are higher near the sea, near mountains and around waterfalls.

Negative ions are said to help people with respiratory disorders by causing particles of dust, pollen, smoke etc. in the air to settle to the ground. An ionizer is a device which emits negative ions into the air. Some models are combined with an air filter.

MASSAGE

Massage has enormous benefits to offer whether you have asthma or not. It is probably the oldest and most instinctive form of therapy known to humanity.

Massage can soothe aches and pains, relieve stress and tension, improve circulation and muscle tone and bring about a wonderful feeling of calm and wellbeing. It also helps to remove toxins from the body's tissues by stimulating the lymphatic system and blood flow. The relaxation provided by massage is vitally important to the person with asthma.

There are several types of massage, including the Chinese acupressure and Japanese Shiatsu, both of which work on the same principle as acupuncture—certain areas of the body are massaged in a certain way to rebalance the body's energy flow.

AROMATHERAPY

Essential oils derived from various plants are used for massage or inhalation in aromatherapy. As the oils are very concentrated, only a very small amount is needed either in hot water for inhaling or added to a base oil for massage. Eucalyptus oil has long been used to clear mucous congestion. Chamomile oil has anti-inflammatory properties and together with bergamot and lavender, it is said to improve immunity. Hyssop oil is said to be an antiseptic and expectorant.

There is a wide range of oils available, each one having special benefits and uses. Many are said to have important psychological as well as physical effects. Studies have proven that different scents affect our moods and sense of wellbeing—in Japan they are even used to improve working efficiency. Some oils, such as citrus, have a stimulating effect, whereas others, like lavender, can help you to relax. Scents affect our feelings because our scent receptors are situated in the part of the brain that registers emotions.

QI GONG AND TAI CHI

Qi gong is a Chinese breathing therapy which has been found to be extremely helpful for a number of health problems, but particularly those affecting the lungs. It is similar in principle to Tai Chi, a series of slow, rhythmical movements combined with breathing exercises which improve the flow of body energy. The movements are often based on those of animals and birds, such as the crane.

BUTEYKO TECHNIQUE

Buteyko technique is a Russian technique for controlling asthma. It involves learning a different pattern of breathing by simple exercises. The technique consists essentially of breath reduction exercises that are aimed at reversing chronic hyperventilation. By correcting the patient's breathing, and normalizing the carbon dioxide in the lung, the body responds in normalizing its metabolism and reducing bronchial spasms. This technique is highly recommended, particularly in those asthmatics who are triggered by exercise, excitement, laughter and emotional trauma.

PROBLEMS COMMONLY
ASSOCIATED WITH ASTHMA:
HAYFEVER, ECZEMA

HAYFEVER (ALLERGIC RHINITIS)

A very high percentage of people with asthma also suffer from allergic rhinitis. This is a medical term used to describe an allergic reaction which primarily affects the nasal passages. Sneezing, excessive nasal mucous, swelling and intense itching of the nasal lining (the itching may also be felt in the ears, throat, and mouth), are the characteristics of allergic rhinitis. Red, itchy, watering, light-sensitive eyes are also a common feature, along with headache, weakness, dizziness and generally feeling unwell.

If severe and long-lasting, this problem can become quite debilitating and cause a great deal of misery. Some people are so severely affected that it undermines their ability to work and to enjoy life. Many chronic sufferers regularly take antihistamine preparations which usually cause significant drowsiness as well as other adverse reactions, and they are often not very effective.

The term 'hayfever' came about as a result of allergic rhinitis occurring in the 'hay season'—or spring and summer when plant pollens are at their peak. Hayfever is generally referred to at these times as allergic rhinitis which is caused by airborne pollens. The symptoms described above can occur at any time of the year and can be triggered by a wide range of antigens or irritants.

Like asthma, allergic rhinitis, (AR), causes an inflammation of mucous membrane which can lead to further complications and chronic symptoms if left untreated. Again, treating the symptoms rather than the cause is useless and can exacerbate the problem. When people ignore their general health and environment, and treat the symptoms when they arise with antihistamines, they are only prolonging their suffering. Chronic irritation and inflammation of the nasal passages can lead to sinusitis, throat and ear infections and nasal polyps—growths in the lining of the nose which are difficult to treat and very uncomfortable as the nose feels as though it is permanently blocked.

Many of the triggers of AR symptoms are the same as those of asthma. Dust and dust mite, animal danders, mold spores, cigarette smoke, pesticides etc. are common precipitating factors. Nasal polyps are frequently caused by a sensitivity to salicylates, and many cases of chronic mucous or catarrh are caused by an allergy to milk or other food. Specific symptoms and causes can vary widely from person to person, but there is no doubt that everyone can benefit from nutritional treatment for their immune system and general health. Much of the information in this book is relevant to the treatment and prevention of allergic rhinitis and other allergies as well as asthma.

The first and sometimes most difficult step in treating and preventing allergic rhinitis is identifying and eliminating the offending allergens or irritants from your environment. Quite often, there is more than one allergen which is causing trouble. Dust mites and pollens (see Chapter 2, Common Triggers of Asthma) do not necessarily have to cause an immune reaction (allergic) to damage mucous membranes and provoke inflammation. They both contain strong irritant substances and should be avoided as much as possible by anyone with symptoms such as those described above. Diesel fumes increase nasal sensitivity to pollens in particular and so should be avoided.

Mold is a very common trigger of AR symptoms and possible sources should be found and treated appropriately. Chapter 6, Practical Help, offers suggestions for dealing with common irritants and allergens such as mold, dust, etc.

Inside the nasal cavity there is a large area of mucous membrane which warms, filters and moistens air as we inhale, protecting our lungs from cold, dry air and particles of dust, etc. Tiny hair-like fibers called cilia, which cover the mucous membrane, help to work the mucous which contains the trapped particles toward the throat where it is swallowed. Keeping this mucous membrane in good condition is obviously extremely important to our health in a number of ways.

Smoking cigarettes and inhaling various corrosive fumes and other substances can destroy or render useless the cilia fibers which are needed to transport harmful particles away from the nasal membrane. If these particles—which may include bacteria and countless other microscopic hazards— are allowed to remain, they are likely to penetrate the mucous membrane, and in the case of bacteria, multiply, setting up inflammation and infection. Once the protective lining of the nose has been worn away or weakened by chronic inflammation, allergic reactions and infections can become increasingly troublesome.

When inflamed, the lining of the nose becomes swollen, mucous production increases, and it becomes difficult for the mucous to drain away. All of this leads to a collection of thickened mucous in the nasal cavity which may create a localized bacterial infection, or, the infection might extend to the nearby sinuses or travel down the eustachian tubes to cause a middle ear infection. A throat infection is also possible as the infected mucous drains down into the lower part of the pharynx. Also, breathing in through the mouth due to a blocked nose means that the lungs have to deal with air which has not been warmed, moistened and filtered, and asthma could be triggered.

SINUSITIS

The sinuses are air-filled cavities in the bones of the face. The nasal cavity is connected to the sinuses by very small openings, and when inflammation or infection spreads into the sinuses from the nasal cavity, sinusitis occurs.

Sinusitis can develop into a very nasty infection, causing quite a degree of illness if left untreated. As well as extreme nasal congestion and a thick, purulent mucous discharge, pain and tenderness is common in the eye area, face and at the front of the head. There may be swollen glands beneath the jaw and possibly a high temperature. Sometimes in very severe infections, the nose and eye area may become swollen and extremely painful. Pressure and sharp pain may also be felt when leaning forward. Allergic rhinitis, viral infections (colds), or any condition, which causes impaired mucous drainage from the nose, can lead to sinusitis.

Quite often congestion and infection can extend to the eustachian tubes —the tubes that lead from the pharynx to the ears—and this can cause fluid to be trapped in the inner ear, affecting hearing and possibly balance. Infection of the middle ear (otitis media) can also occur as a complication of this. In children, the adenoids are a common contributing factor to middle ear infections as they can become swollen due to nasal, sinus or throat inflammation, and block the eustachian tubes.

Aspirin sensitivity is found in one third of patients having nasal polyps, rhinosinusitis and asthma. Individuals with nasal polyps have high level of platelet activating factor (PAF) in the polyp. Irritation of polyps can give release to PAF resulting in mucus discharge and edema.

Treatment involves re-establishing drainage and clearing up any infection. This can be done by the use of antibiotics, improving the rheology of mucus by thinning it (by using N-acetylcysteine, garlic, horseradish or papain) and decongesting edematous membranes with quercetin.

An unrecognized cause of sinusitis can be gastroesphageal reflux (GEPR). Many studies have shown that the incidence of GEPR is much higher in patients with chronic sinusitis who do not respond to conventional treatment.

TREATMENT AND PREVENTION

◆ Identify and avoid allergens and irritants. Follow the guidelines in Chapter 6 for creating a healthy environment. It may be necessary to use an elimination diet to determine which dietary factors are involved. Cow's milk sensitivity is a common problem. Milk increases nasal mucous in many people. The elimination diet also acts as a cleansing program to remove toxins and waste build-up in the body. This is very important to the body's natural healing processes.

- Correct any nutritional deficiencies (see Chapter 4).
- Check for salicylate sensitivity, especially if nasal polyps are present (see Chapter 9—Salicylate Content).
- If a known sensitivity to ragweed exists, you may need to avoid zucchini, cucumber, banana, rockmelon, watermelon and honeydew melon. All of these foods share a common allergen with ragweed.
- Sugar, white flour and all refined carbohydrates should be avoided, as these substances are known to aggravate conditions where mucous is a problem. It is interesting to note that grass pollens, which are common causes of hayfever, cane sugar and wheat, are all in the same botanical family of grasses.
- Rinsing the mouth, throat, nose and eyes with saline will help to remove allergenic particles and will also help to clear mucous. Hydrastis (Golden Seal) tea is also very good for rinsing the nose, especially in treating sinusitis.
- Steam inhalations (using a bowl of hot water or a vaporizer) are very helpful for clearing congestion. A few drops of Olbas™ oil can relieve symptoms of hayfever, and eucalyptus or menthol is very good for clearing congestion. Eucalyptus and menthol can also be used in packs (try a face washer wrung out in hot water that has had a few drops of oil added to it) and applied to the sinus area to relieve pressure and pain.
- Vitamin C and magnesium are natural antihistamines, and many people have had relief from hayfever symptoms by taking pantothenic acid (Vitamin B5). Bioflavonoids are also important for reducing the inflammatory and allergic reaction. The bioflavonoid quercetin reduces tissue swelling and congestion as well as reduces nasal polyp formation.
- Fenugreek tea is very helpful for sinusitis. Two cups per day is recommended.
- Apply a hot pack over the sinus area.
- Suck zinc gluconate lozenges (50 mg).
- Include plenty of garlic, onions and horseradish in the diet, or use immune-enhancing supplements.

◆ To improve immunity, supplement with fish oil (cod liver oil is beneficial as it also contains vitamins A and D —very important nutrients for healthy mucous membrane), zinc, vitamin C (at least 1500 mg. per day) and antioxidant nutrients (see Chapter 4 for further information on nutrients). The enzyme bromelain (used in digestive enzyme formula) can be very helpful in allergic and inflammatory conditions as it inhibits inflammatory processes in the body.

◆ Taking beeswax may decrease sensitization to pollens.

◆ Avoid exposure to diesel fumes as it sensitizes the nose to pollens. Oxides of nitrogen can destroy cilia in the throat and hence encourage the accumulation of mucus.

◆ Treat gastroesophagel reflux with a fiber and acid supplement. Vinegar in water with meals may be sufficient to improve stomach acidity.

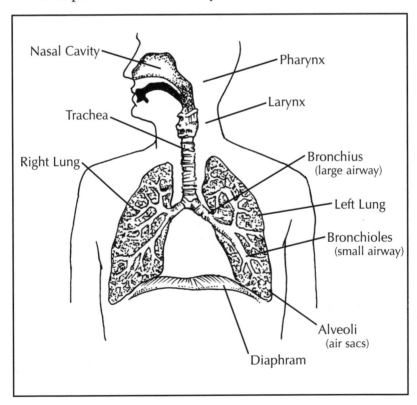

ECZEMA AND URTICARIA (HIVES)

Allergy-prone individuals often tend to have 'sensitive skin,' developing dermatitis or eczema of one form or another quite frequently. They may react to a number of external irritants such as detergents and other chemicals, or their condition may be directly linked to food allergy or nutritional deficiencies. A wide range of things, including emotional stress may trigger urticaria. Quite often, too much emphasis is placed on treating skin conditions externally with creams and ointments, when the basis of the problem is actually internal.

There is a **very high incidence of eczema among asthma sufferers, particularly children**. A specific group of inflammatory mediators are responsible for the connection between the two conditions—leukotrienes. These mediators appear to be linked to excessive production of the pro-inflammatory prostaglandins, caused by faulty essential fatty acid metabolism and a deficiency in zinc, vitamin C, B3 and B6. Vitamin E, and quercetin inhibits or modulates the synthesis of leukotrienes. A great many cases of eczema have cleared up after supplements of essential fatty acids were taken. Hydrochloric acid deficiency is common among chronic eczema sufferers (this is also common among asthma sufferers), particularly children. This deficiency is associated with low levels of the B group vitamins and possibly mercury amalgam dental fillings.

The presentation of any of the above skin conditions can vary greatly and diagnosis is sometimes difficult. Atopic (allergic) eczema can appear as dry, rough inflamed patches or as areas of small, weeping pustules. Common areas of the body affected are the upper back and shoulders, inside the elbows and knees and sometimes the face, but it can vary from person to person. Eczema is always characterized by itching, and secondary infections can occur in severe cases as a result of scratching.

Eczema often appears in babies shortly after the cessation of breastfeeding or the introduction of solid foods, making the cause of the problem fairly clear. Milk, wheat and eggs are the most common foods known to cause eczema, especially in babies and children, and many cases have cleared up completely after the offending food—usually cow's milk—has been discontinued.

Contact dermatitis can be caused by a number of substances, some of the most common are: cosmetics, hair colors, perfumes, soaps, detergents (detergent residue on clothes is a common problem) and a number of other chemicals. Skin contact with certain foods and pesticide residues can also cause quite severe reactions in some people; peach skin is a common irritant in this way.

Urticaria (hives) often appears as a rather dramatic red rash which may have small white lumps and is intensely itchy. It may occur suddenly as a reaction to a food, emotional stress or direct skin contact with an allergenic substance. Sometimes, hives may resemble insect bites—a number of intensely itchy red lumps may develop and then disappear within a few hours. Severe hives may occur along with tissue swelling in very serious allergic reactions. Salicylates, aspirin and food additives, particularly tartrazine, are common causes of hives.

PREVENTION AND TREATMENT

- Identify and avoid any foods, chemicals, etc. which may be causing symptoms. An elimination diet may be needed (See Chapter 9).
- DON'T scratch.
- Be careful in the sun, particularly if skin is inflamed as it may aggravate the condition.
- Don't allow skin to become dry but be wary of creams and moisturizers; some may make the problem worse. Use plain Sorbelene cream (contains glycerol and cetomacrogol) or refer to the products recommended in this book.
- Soap is very drying and often contains irritant substances Sorbelene can be used as a soap substitute.
- Essential fatty acid supplements are **vitally important** i.e. fish oils and evening primrose oil (See Chapter 4). Also, ensure adequate intake of zinc, vitamins A, D, C, B

group, E and all antioxidant nutrients. Bioflavonoids will help to combat inflammation.

◆ Improve digestion with digestive enzyme supplements (See recommended products list).

◆ For acute contact dermatitis reactions, apply ice cold compresses using white cotton fabric for half an hour several times a day.

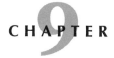

CHAPTER

DIETARY GUIDELINES

Asthma is just one of many conditions which may be caused or aggravated by a sensitivity to foods and food additives. Rhinitis, eczema, hives, headaches, gastrointestinal problems and hyperactivity are some of the problems commonly associated with food allergy and intolerance.

It is often difficult to determine which foods are causing adverse reactions without the use of an elimination diet. Keeping a food-symptom diary for a few weeks can sometimes be helpful, but because reactions often vary in the time they take to occur as well as in severity, the full elimination diet may be necessary to provide conclusive information.

POINTS TO CONSIDER

◆ A suspected food may not always cause a reaction, or, the reaction may vary in severity. This depends on the amount consumed, the condition or ripeness of the food, the way in which the food is prepared (raw, cooked etc.), what other foods are eaten at the same time (some may alter the digestion process), and possibly, the use of medications which contain antihistamines (this could mask symptoms).

◆ Foods may contain a variety of substances, which may cause a reaction similar in effect to food allergy. Mold, additives, pesticides, bacteria and various other toxins may contaminate food and cause symptoms.

◆ Clear results are more easily obtained with the elimination diet when only a few foods cause symptoms. When there is a large number of allergens involved, it may take longer to determine specific causes and effects.

◆ Adverse reactions to foods are more likely to occur if there is a deficiency in certain nutrients, digestive problems are present or if excessive amounts of certain foods are being consumed (such as salt, sugar or alcohol).

◆ When starting an elimination diet, all medication should be taken into account in as much as many preparations contain additives. Nutritional supplements should also be approved by your physician/nutritionist as being free of potential allergens.

◆ The elimination diet, which is followed by reintroducing suspect foods, should only be used when symptoms are not life-threatening.

◆ Some people may experience a worsening of certain symptoms in the first few days on the diet. This 'withdrawal' phase may last up to 8 days but symptoms should have subsided by day 12. On rare occasions, one of the foods allowed may cause a reaction in some individuals.

◆ It may take two days or up to two weeks before improvement is obvious on the diet.

◆ An elimination diet must be followed carefully and thoroughly if it is to provide clear results. Professional guidance may be needed, particularly for children or those who have severe symptoms. A dietitian or physician who specializes in nutrition and allergy should be consulted —most GPs do not have specialist knowledge of nutrition. It is important to ensure that nutritional intake is adequate when on a restricted diet.

ROTATIONAL FULL ELIMINATION DIET

The purpose of this diet is to eliminate all of the common food and chemical allergens for a period of 12 to 16 days, followed by a 'challenge' period to determine specific sensitivities.

During the challenge period each food being tested is eaten for at least three days. Symptoms are recorded during this period. If no reaction occurs, this food may remain in the diet and the next food can now be tested. If symptoms do occur, however, this food should again be avoided and the next food should not be tested for at least two days. Remember, an adverse reaction can occur almost immediately or it can take hours or even days, depending on the amount consumed and individual tolerance level.

(Do not attempt this rotation diet without medical supervision. The withdrawal and challenge phase of this diet may bring on severe symptoms in some individuals.)

THE ELIMINATION PHASE

The foods given in the following lists may be eaten at any time and in any combination provided only the foods listed for that day are eaten, i.e. foods listed on one day cannot be mixed or changed with foods from another day unless testing has proven that they are non-reactive to the individual. All foods other than those listed here must be strictly avoided. Coffee and tea, of course, are not allowed, but for those who regularly consume large amounts of either, it may be necessary to remove them gradually. Sudden withdrawal of caffeine can cause a number of unpleasant symptoms, including a possible aggravation of asthma, as the drug theophylline is provided by coffee. Theophylline is a bronchodilator which is taken as an oral medication (Refer Chapter 3—Medical Treatment of Asthma).

The following food lists form the basis of the elimination diet. Once the first four days of the diet have been followed, simply start at day 1 again and repeat the routine for a total of at least 12 days. Some people may need to follow the diet for 16 days to be free of symptoms.

DAY 1
Sweet Potato (peeled)
Pears (peeled)
Veal or Rabbit
Chicken or Turkey

DAY 2
Rice
Lemon
Papaya

DAY 3
Tapioca
Delicious Apples (peeled)
Whiting or BreamBuckwheat
Tuna

DAY 4
Sago
Lamb
Bananas (Cavendish)

Vegetarians may substitute dried peas and red or brown lentils for any animal protein listed.

In addition to the foods listed above, the following may be added at any time:

Puffed millet, millet flour, rice cakes and wafers, rice crispbread, cashews, cashew paste, lettuce, celery, cabbage, bamboo shoots and turnip.

Restrict to half a cup: green beans, red cabbage, brussel sprouts, mung bean sprouts, green peas, leeks, choko, shallots and chives.

Restrict to one tablespoon per serving: sweet potato, broccoli, parsnip, carrot, beetroot, spinach, onion, cauliflower, pumpkin, asparagus and turnip. Cold pressed sunflower, safflower and flax oil may be used for salad dressings etc. Salt, garlic and parsley are allowed and a small amount of olive oil may be used for cooking. Butter and margarine are NOT allowed.

All vegetables MUST be washed and peeled before cooking.

All water must be either boiled or filtered before use. Plain mineral or soda water and fresh pear juice may be used as desired.

Medications often contain colors and other additives. A doctor should be consulted about contents of these and suitable alternatives should be found. With colored capsules, the contents may be emptied and taken and the gelatin capsule discarded. Colored tablets may sometimes be washed under the tap to remove colored coating. Check with a doctor first. Colored elixirs such as children's Panadol™ (always keep out of reach of children) are best avoided—instead, try crushing appropriate dosage portion of a Panadol™ (paracetamol) tablet and mix into golden syrup. Panadol™ taken with a hot drink is a good alternative to cough mixtures and will soothe the throat. Aspirin-based drugs should be avoided.

Injected medications may contain preservatives, and sensitive individuals should discuss possible alternatives with their doctor.

Constipation may be treated with psyllium or rice bran and plenty of water should be taken. Unflavored fiber preparations may also be taken. For severe diarrhea, abdominal pain or any other complaints, a suitable unflavored, uncolored medication could be obtained from your doctor, if necessary.

THE CHALLENGE PHASE

Foods may be tested in any order, but it is recommended that foods that are missed most are tested first. Dairy products, wheat, salicylates and natural colors should be tested before other foods as these food groups form a major part of most diets.

If no reaction occurs after testing a food for three days, continue to use that food and go on to the next challenge. If symptoms do occur, however, remove that food group immediately and wait until symptoms have subsided before testing another food (usually 2 or 3 days).

All foods must be tested within each group before a decision is made about which foods are responsible for symptoms.

This food rotation and challenge program should be performed during periods of low social activity as there is a possibility of sickness occurring. Any pre-existing infection may increase the severity of symptoms.

METHOD OF CHALLENGING

- **Dairy Foods**—Have three glasses of milk per day for three days. If no reaction occurs, try natural yogurt, cheese and other dairy products.
- **Wheat and grains**—Three whole wheat crackers per day with milk (if milk has been proven safe) or pear juice, or scones made without milk or yeast. Other grains to be tested in order are oats, barley and rye.
- **Egg and egg products**—Egg white should be eaten in small quantities throughout the day, (egg yolk can be tested after this).
- **Yeast**—One teaspoon per day of food yeast or other yeast extract for three days.
- **Salicylates**—Drink four glasses of orange or tomato juice with no added preservatives or colors.

- ◆ **Preservatives and artificial colors**—Eat large amounts of colored lollipops, jubes etc.
- ◆ **Seafood**—Shell fish and mullet should be tried in small amounts.
- ◆ **Alcohol**—Test beer, wine and spirits.
- ◆ **Tap water**—Take three large glasses.
- ◆ **Cane sugar**—One tablespoon dissolved in warm water and added to one cup of pear juice.
- • **Beef**—ground, steak or roast.

It is important to remember that when testing foods, all symptoms must be recorded and only the foods listed should be eaten along with the food being tested. Do not add any other foods.

SYMPTOMS TO LOOK FOR WHEN TESTING FOODS

Joints	Aches and pains, stiffness, swelling, redness or warmth in the joint area.
Skin	Itching, hives, flushing, pallor, sweating, and rashes.
Head	Headache, migraine, a feeling of pressure or tightness, a throbbing or stabbing sensation.
Fatigue	Tiredness, yawning, a feeling of heaviness or exhaustion, falling asleep.
Muscle	Tremor, jerking, cramps, spasm or weakness.
Nasal	Sneezing, itchy nose, discharge, post-nasal drip, congestion, sinus discomfort.
Mouth, Throat	Soreness, tightness, swelling, difficulty in swallowing, hoarseness, metallic or bad taste in the mouth, excess saliva.
Ears	Blocked ears, itching, earache, ringing in the ears, hearing loss, sensitivity to noise.
Eyes	Itching, burning, tearing, redness, swelling (allergic shiner), heavy feeling. Blurred or double vision, flashes, vision loss, sensitivity to light.

Lungs, Heart	Coughing, wheezing, heaviness or tightness in the chest, rapid breathing, chest pain, rapid pulse, palpitations, irregular heartbeat.
Kidney	Mild urge to urinate, painful or difficult urination, genital itch.
Digestive System	Nausea, belching, vomiting, a bloated or full feeling, diarrhea, constipation, unusual hunger or thirst, heartburn, abdominal pain.
Other	Dizziness, lightheadedness, loss of balance, vertigo, chills or hot flushes, bedwetting.
Neurological Symptoms	Food or chemical sensitivity can affect the brain and central nervous system in the following ways. The individual may be:
Depressed	withdrawn, listless, vacant, indifferent, confused, dazed, crying.
Stimulated	talkative, hyperactive, silly, intoxicated, tense, restless, anxious, afraid, irritable or angry.

Vitamin C and bicarb of soda (or Alkali—see recommended product list) can be very helpful for reducing severity of adverse reactions.

SAMPLE MENUS FOR ELIMINATION DIET

DAY 1

Breakfast
- ◆ Boiled millet and pear juice
- ◆ Rice wafers or cakes with cashew paste

Lunch
- ◆ Coleslaw with cashews

Dinner
- ◆ Roast veal — garlic and salt may be used
- ◆ Roast sweet potato
- ◆ Steamed brussel sprouts
- ◆ Green peas

DAY 2

Breakfast
- • Papaya with a sprinkle of lemon juice
- • Rice wafers with cashew paste

Lunch
- • Salad—lettuce, chives, cashews, sunflower oil
- • Rice wafers and cashew paste

Dinner
- Roast Chicken with Rice stuffing (see recipes)
- Cabbage with Mung Beans (see recipes
- Papaya and lemon juice

DAY 3

Breakfast
- Boiled brown rice with freshly pureed delicious apple
- Rice wafer with cashew paste

Lunch
- Tuna in oil
- Salad using allowed foods
- Peeled sliced apples

Dinner
- Grilled Whole Bream (see recipes)
- Lettuce and Mung Beans
- Rice wafers
- Tapioca in Pear juice (see recipes)

DAY 4

Breakfast
- Sago in Pear juice (see recipes)

Lunch
- Cold sliced lamb
- Buckwheat Tabhouli (see recipes)
- Tossed salad (see recipes)

Dinner
- Lamb Kebabs (see recipes)
- Tossed salad
- Sago with Pear and Banana cream (see recipes)

RECIPES FOR ELIMINATION DIET

Buckwheat Tabhouli

1 cup buckwheat grits (soak for 30 minutes)
1 cup shallots, chopped
½ cup continental parsley, chopped
1 cup celery, finely chopped
¼ cup sunflower or safflower oil
1 large clove garlic, minced
2 tablespoons onion, finely chopped
Juice of ½ lemon, salt to taste

Drain buckwheat thoroughly, add other ingredients and mix well.

Roast Chicken with Rice Stuffing

Wash, drain and remove fat from a free-range chicken.

Stuffing
1 cup brown rice
1 cup shallots, chopped
1 dessertspoon oil
1 large clove garlic, minced
3 tablespoons parsley, chopped

Boil rice in salted water for 30 minutes, drain. Sauté remaining ingredients gently then add to rice and mix well. Stuff chicken with mixture in place in baking dish with ½ cup water. Bake in moderate oven until cooked.

Cabbage with Mung Beans

¼ medium cabbage
1 cup green beans, chopped
1 tablespoon olive oil (if salicylates not a problem)
1 cup celery, chopped
1 large clove garlic, minced
1 leek, finely sliced
1 cup filtered water
1 cup mung bean sprouts

Place all ingredients except bean sprouts in a pot and cook gently until tender. Add bean sprouts for final minute of cooking time.

Lettuce and Mung Bean Salad

1 lettuce
1 cup celery, chopped
1 cup mung bean sprouts
2 tablespoons onion, finely sliced

Toss ingredients together with a little sunflower oil and lemon juice.

Grilled Whole Bream

4 whole bream, cleaned and scaled
2 large cloves garlic, minced
2 tablespoons olive oil (if salicylates are not a problem)

1 cup shallots, sliced diagonally
1 tablespoon parsley, chopped

Wash fish and pat dry. Place half the garlic and half the olive oil inside the fish—make slits on both sides of fish to do this. Place under grill and cook until flesh flakes easily. Meanwhile, sauté remaining ingredients and place decoratively over fish before serving.

Coleslaw

2 cups shredded cabbage
2 shallots, chopped
2–3 tablespoons parsley, chopped
½ small carrot grated
½ onion, finely sliced
½ cup mung bean sprouts

Toss together with ¼ cup sunflower oil and juice of ½ lemon.

Lamb Kebabs—Greek Style

1¼ lb. lamb fillet, fat removed
2 large cloves garlic
chopped parsley
1 tablespoon lemon juice
1 tablespoon olive oil

Cut fillets into 4 cm cubes. Marinate for 2 hours in remaining ingredients. Thread onto bamboo skewers which have been soaked in water for 1 hour. Grill, brushing with marinade occasionally.

Sago in Pear Juice

1 cup sago
2 large pears, pureed with 1 cup water

Cook sago slowly in pear puree and water, stirring often. Add some hot water if the mixture becomes too thick—up to 2 cups extra water may be needed. The sago is cooked when it is clear (cooking time is reduced if sago is soaked overnight first). Use the same method for TAPIOCA IN PEAR JUICE (some lemon juice may also be added). Serve hot for breakfast or chilled for desert.

Sago with Pear and Banana Cream

Puree one pear and 2 bananas and serve with chilled sago.

LIVING WITH FOOD SENSITIVITIES

The following dietary suggestions are for people with a proven sensitivity to some of the common food antigens—wheat, milk and egg, etc. For lists of foods containing sulfites, MSG, etc. see Chapter 4—Dangers in our Diet.

MILK-FREE DIET

The following must be avoided: milk, buttermilk, cream, sour cream, ice-cream, butter, custards, cream sauces, soups and any other foods containing cow's milk or casein protein. Many processed foods contain milk products, and most margarine also contains milk solids. All labels should be checked.

Finding substitutes for cow's milk is becoming easier. There are many good products made using soy bean milk or rice, including tofu or rice-based ice cream. Goat's milk is not always a viable alternative as it may still cause a reaction in some people and it often has a very strong taste. Sheep's milk is less readily available, but it does have a more pleasant taste and is less likely to cause a reaction. Coconut cream or milk can be used for some recipes. Almond, sesame or cashew 'milk' and cream can be made and these are quite nutritious.

Clarified butter (ghee) can sometimes be tolerated as most of the milk proteins are removed during processing. This can be made at home by melting butter over a low heat, allowing it to cool a little and carefully pouring it into a glass jar. Most of the proteins will settle in the bottom of the pan or the jar and are obvious as small white particles. Keep clarified butter in the fridge. Tahini—ground sesame seeds—and sunflower spread are healthy alternatives to butter, but tahini should not be eaten in excessive amounts. Soy butter is now available and there are some milk-free brands of margarine available.

Soy-based cheese is often available, and Greek feta cheese made from sheep's milk is also a very well-tolerated alternative to cheese made from cow's milk.

It is very important that alternative sources are found for the nutrients normally provided by cow's milk. In the U.S., cow's milk is a major source of protein and calcium as well as a number of vitamins and minerals, especially vitamins A and D. Vitamin D is important for the absorption of calcium, and vitamin A is necessary for the immune system and for healthy mucous membranes. See Chapter 4 for other rich sources of these nutrients. Many people on milk-free diets will require supplements, particularly of the nutrients mentioned above.

WHEAT-FREE DIET

This diet can be difficult to begin with as most people in western societies eat very large amounts of this grain in a wide variety of foods. The following must be avoided: bread of all kinds unless free of all forms of wheat and gluten, waffles, wheat-based cereals such as Weet bix or semolina, pancakes, pastry, cakes, scones, muffins, bagels, pies, biscuits, crumbed foods, sausages, pasta, pretzels, and any other food which contains wheat flour or starch. A large variety of packet or processed foods do contain wheat in some form, but at least it is now possible to check ingredients on labels.

There is now a large variety of products available for people on wheat-free diets. Pasta made from rice, corn and buckwheat is available from healthfood shops. Gluten-free bread is available from some shops, or prepared mixes can be bought to make the bread yourself. Rice flour, maize (corn) flour, potato flour, soy flour and others are available for use in many recipes. Rice cakes, rice crispbread and rice wafers are readily available in supermarkets, and rice cookies and crackers can also be found in healthfood shops. Plain popcorn and plain potato chips (made using only salt and oil) are quite healthy snacks also. It may take a little time, but quite a few tasty alternatives can be found to the usual wheat-based foods.

It is possible that a sensitivity to rye, oats and barley will exist along with a wheat sensitivity. If so, beer and whiskey will need to be avoided.

Other probably safe wheat substitutes include: sago,

tapioca, millet, graham flour (perhaps), lentil flour, polenta, wild rice and chickpea flour.

EGGS

Sometimes allergy is restricted to the white of the egg, and so, the yolk can be used for many recipes. When the whole egg must be avoided, there are several substitutes. Gelatin can be used where egg is normally used to 'set' puddings such as custard. One teaspoon of gelatin dissolved in a little hot water is roughly equivalent to one egg. In biscuit recipes, one egg can be replaced by 2 tablespoons water, 1 tablespoon vegetable oil and ½ teaspoon baking powder.

CHOCOLATE

Carob makes a reasonable substitute for chocolate. Health food shops have a variety of carob products and it is also possible to buy carob powder for cooking.

METABISULPHITE (Preservative)

LOW META BISULPHITE DIET FOR ASTHMA SUFFERERS

Avoid: All dried fruits (with SO2), preserved fruit juices, brewed products—wine, preserved cider, beer, dried vegetables, instant potato, uncooked prawns, cordials, soft drinks, dessert toppings, flavoring essences, cheese spreads, cheese pastes, bread with dried fruits, fruit cake, marzipan, cereals containing dried fruits, muesli, hot chips, pickles, pickled onion, chutney, pickled or corn meats, tomato sauce, roll mops, commercial salad dressings, chocolates.

BENZOIC ACID (Preservative)

Avoid: Soft drinks, cider, cordials, fruit juice drink, fruit drink, preserved fruit juice, fruit flavored drinks, flavored toppings, fruit juice syrup, liquid essences, fish marinades, preserved cherries, imitation fruit, low-joule jam, berries, prunes, plums, cinnamon, cloves.

TARTRAZINE (Yellow coloring)

Occurs in: Some breakfast cereals, some lollipops, colored ice-cream and sherbets, gelatin desserts, packet dessert toppings, orange flavored drink mixes, soft drinks, fruit juice cordial, mint sauce and jelly, colored icing, some margarine, some cheese products, some medications, marzipan, pickles, canned peas, brown sauce. Other phenolic compounds that may activate the inflammatory response are: vanillin, eugenol, propylgallate propylparaben, butylated hydroxy-anisole (BHA) butylated hydroxy toluine (BHT), aspartame (Nutrasweet™).

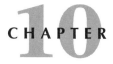

CHAPTER

RECIPES

Recipes are marked **E** if egg free, **W** if wheat free, and **M** if milk free. There are a number of delicious vegetarian dishes included. All recipes are highly nutritious, based on fresh ingredients and additive free.

Guacomole   E W M
2 ripe avocados, mashed
1 small onion, finely chopped
1 clove garlic, minced
2 ripe tomatoes, finely chopped
minced chili to taste
1 small capsicum, finely chopped
½ cup finely chopped celery

Combine all ingredients and mix well. Serve with wheat-free corn chips or rice crackers.

Hummus   E W M
2/3 lb. cooked, drained chickpeas
2 dessertspoons olive oil
2 tablespoons tahini (sesame seed paste)
1 clove garlic, minced
2 dessertspoons lemon juice
pinch of salt

Combine ingredients and mash well. Sprinkle with a little paprika. This makes a very good dip or spread.

Minestrone   E W M
¼ cup haricot, kidney or black-eyed beans, soaked overnight
1 onion, chopped
2 cloves garlic, minced
1 cup chopped celery
1 leek, sliced

1 tablespoon olive oil
1 large potato, diced
1 cup chopped carrot
½ cup green beans, chopped
1 cup chopped broccoli or cabbage
1 teaspoon miso (available from health food shops)
25 oz. water
1 small tomato, finely chopped
½ teaspoon fresh basil
salt and pepper to taste

Boil beans rapidly for 10 minutes, then simmer for 35 minutes. Fry onion, garlic, leek and celery in olive oil. Add all other ingredients, bring to the boil, and then simmer for 20 minutes.

Leek and Potato Soup   E W M

1 lb. leeks, sliced
1 onion, chopped
1 lb. potatoes, peeled and sliced
½ quart chicken or vegetable stock
½ quart soy or rice milk
fresh parsley
salt, pepper to taste

Boil vegetables and stock together until vegetables are tender. Press through a large sieve or process in a blender. Pour puree back into saucepan, add soy milk, season and serve.

Ratatouille   E W M

1 onion, chopped
2 cloves garlic, minced
1 tablespoon olive oil
1 cup chopped celery
1 leek, sliced
2 carrots, sliced
1 large zucchini, sliced
3 large, ripe tomatoes, skinned and finely chopped
salt and pepper to taste

Sauté onion and garlic in oil. Add other vegetables and cook for about 15 minutes. Season to taste and serve.

Seafood Risotto   E W M

1 onion, chopped
1 clove garlic, minced
1 tablespoon olive oil
1 small green pepper, chopped
1/8 lb. mushrooms, sliced
½ quart chicken or vegetable stock
½ lb. g rice
fresh parsley, chopped
¼ lb. shrimp, cooked
¼ lb. crab meat

Sauté onion and garlic in oil, add pepper and mushrooms, and cook gently for 2 minutes. Add stock and rice, boil gently until rice is cooked and all liquid is absorbed. Stir in prawns and crabmeat and heat through. Sprinkle with parsley and serve.

Sate Chicken   E W M

2¼ lb. chicken thigh fillets
1 onion, finely chopped
2 cloves garlic, minced
1 teaspoon cumin powder
1 teaspoon minced ginger
1 teaspoon curry powder
1 tablespoon soy sauce
  (check that you are using an MSG-free brand)
2 tablespoons lemon juice
1–3 hot chilies, minced
½ cup peanut butter
½ cup chopped peanuts or cashews
1 tablespoon honey
1 cup coconut milk

Cut chicken into ¼–1/3" cubes. Marinate in soy sauce, lemon juice, honey, cumin, chilies and coconut milk for at least 2 hours. Sauté onion and garlic in a little olive oil, add drained marinade from chicken and other ingredients, and simmer gently for about 15 minutes while preparing sates. Thread chicken onto bamboo skewers and grill 5 minutes on each side. Serve with sauce poured over. Garnish with sliced cucumber, thin strips of carrot and shallots. Brown Coriander Rice is ideal with this dish.

Lemon Parsley Rice   E W M

4 cups cooked, hot brown rice
4 tablespoons lemon juice
4 tablespoons chopped parsley
4 teaspoons grated lemon rind

Combine ingredients and serve.

Coriander Rice   E W M

4 cups cooked, hot rice
4 tablespoons lemon juice
1 cup finely chopped red bell pepper
4 tablespoons fresh, chopped coriander leaves

Combine all ingredients and serve.

Savory Millet   E W M

1 cup hulled millet
2 cups V8 vegetable juice
1 cup water
½ cup chopped shallots
1 clove garlic, minced
1 teaspoon curry powder

Bring juice and water to the boil in a large pot, add millet and curry powder and garlic. Simmer, covered for 20–25 minutes. Stir in shallots and serve with steamed vegetables.

Ginger Chicken and Vegetables (Chinese style)   E W M

1¼ lb. chicken breast, fat removed
2 tablespoons minced ginger root
3 tablespoons soy sauce (MSG-free brand)
1 tablespoon lemon juice
1 large onion, chopped
4 cloves garlic, minced
1 tablespoon olive oil
2 cups unsweetened pineapple juice
1 red bell pepper, cut into strips
1 green pepper, cut into strips

1 zucchini, cut into strips
2 tablespoons wheat-free corn flour
2 tablespoons water
2 cups mung bean sprouts
1 cup snow peas
½ cup shallots, sliced diagonally
few drops of sesame oil

Cut chicken into small pieces and marinate in ginger, garlic, soy sauce and lemon juice for at least 3 hours. Using a large pan or wok, sauté onion in oil for 1 minute, add chicken and stir fry for 4–5 minutes. Add capsicums and zucchini and cook for another 2–3 minutes. Add juice and heat through. Mix corn flour and water to a smooth paste and add to pan stirring constantly until sauce has thickened. Add sprouts and snow peas and cook for 1 minute. Stir in sesame oil. Garnish with shallots and serve with Lemon Parsley Rice or rice noodles. For variety, use orange juice and broccoli instead of pineapple juice and zucchini.

Ginger Salad   E W M

1 small lettuce, shredded
1 small onion, sliced thinly
1 large carrot, coarsely grated
1 zucchini, grated
2 sticks celery, chopped
¼ cup lemon juice
¼ cup safflower oil
1 tablespoon honey
1 teaspoon minced green ginger

Place juice, oil, honey and ginger into a screw top jar and shake well. Combine vegetables in a large bowl, add dressing and toss well.

Lamb Biriani   E W M

1 tablespoon olive oil
½ cup sliced almonds
1¾ lb. chopped leftover roast lamb
1 onion, chopped
2 cloves garlic, minced

½ teaspoon grated ginger
1-2 chilies, minced (optional)
4 whole cloves
4 cardamom pods
1 teaspoon ground cumin seeds
½ teaspoon turmeric
1 teaspoon ground cinnamon
1 cup brown rice
4 cups beef stock
½ cup chopped raisins

Using a large pan, sauté almonds in oil until golden brown, remove and drain. Add onion, garlic, ginger and spices to hot oil and fry for a few minutes. Add rice and beef stock and simmer for 30 minutes. Add lamb and raisins and simmer for a further 10 minutes. Garnish with almonds and serve with Curried Vegetables, Tomato Sambal, sliced banana and desiccated coconut, and, if milk is allowed, cucumber and yogurt.

Curried Vegetables   E W M

1 tablespoon olive oil or ghee
2 onions, sliced
2 cloves garlic, minced
½ teaspoon grated green ginger
2 teaspoons curry powder
½ teaspoon turmeric
1 teaspoon cumin
½ cauliflower, cut into small pieces
3 potatoes, diced
3 zucchinis, sliced thickly
2 carrots, sliced diagonally
2 tomatoes
½ cup chicken stock
1 tablespoon lemon juice

Sauté onion, garlic and ginger until transparent, add spices and mix in well. Add vegetables, sauté for 2–3 minutes, then add stock and simmer for 10–15 minutes. Stir lemon juice through and serve.

Tomato Sambal   E W M

2 small tomatoes, not too ripe, chopped
2 granny smith apples, chopped
1 cup shallots, chopped
1 tablespoon chopped fresh or dried mint
1 teaspoon raw sugar dissolved in
1 tablespoon vinegar

Combine ingredients and mix well. Serve as an accompaniment to curries.

Tahitian Chicken   E W

2¼ lb. chicken breast fillets
butter for frying
1 cup dry shredded coconut
2 small granny smith apples, sliced
2 medium bananas, sliced
1 teaspoon curry powder
1 cup chicken stock
½ cup cream (or rice, soy or almond milk)

Cut fillets into quarters and flatten slightly. Coat with coconut and fry in butter until golden brown, drain. In a clean pan, sauté apple in a little butter until tender, add curry powder and mix in well. Add banana and stock and simmer for 5 minutes, stir in cream and heat through. Serve with rice and vegetables of choice.

Bali Meatballs   M W

1¼ lb. ground beef
1 large carrot, grated finely
1 teaspoon honey
2 teaspoons soy sauce
1 teaspoon cumin
1 teaspoon curry powder
1 onion, minced
2 cloves garlic, minced
½ cup chopped cashews
1 potato, boiled, drained and mashed
1 egg

Combine all ingredients and mix well, Cover and refrigerate for 1–2 hours. Form mixture into balls and fry in a little olive oil until cooked through. Serve with Peanut Sauce and rice.

Peanut Sauce   E W M

1 onion, chopped
1 clove garlic, minced
½ teaspoon grated ginger
1 teaspoon curry powder
1 teaspoon cumin
1 teaspoon chili pepper, minced
½ cup peanut butter
1 tablespoon soy sauce (MSG-free brand)
1 tablespoon honey
1 tablespoon lemon juice
1 cup coconut milk

Sauté onion, garlic and ginger in a little olive oil, add spices and mix well, cook for 2–3 minutes. Add peanut butter and other ingredients, stirring constantly until well blended. Simmer gently for 15 minutes, stirring frequently. Serve. (Water may be added if sauce is too thick.) If allergic to peanuts, cashew butter may be used.

Salmon Rissoles   W M   (high in calcium)

1 large can salmon, drained well and mashed
1¼ lb. potatoes, peeled, boiled and mashed well
1 large onion, chopped finely
1 egg
1 cup buckwheat flour
olive oil for frying

Combine salmon, potato, onion and egg and mix well. Form into rissoles and coat with buckwheat flour. Fry in a little oil until golden brown.
Serve with Rice Salad.

Rice Salad   E W M

3 cups cooked brown rice, chilled
1 cup chopped shallots
1 cup chopped celery

1 cup chopped red bell pepper
1 carrot, grated
½ cup unsweetened pineapple pieces
1 teaspoon curry powder
¼ cup lemon juice
¼ cup safflower oil
orange slices and chopped parsley to garnish

Combine all ingredients and mix well.

Chicken Salad E W M

1¼ lb. cooked, chopped chicken, all fat removed
1 large zucchini, grated
2 medium carrots, grated
1 medium beet, peeled and grated
1 large apple, grated
¼ cup lemon juice
1 cup chopped shallots
1 large stick celery, finely chopped
2 tomatoes, chopped
1 cup mung bean sprouts
¼ bunch watercress, chopped

Stir lemon juice into grated apple, mix with other ingredients. Garnish with extra watercress leaves and a sprinkle of sesame seeds.

Chicken Yakatori E W M

2¼ lb. chicken thigh fillets
1 bunch shallots
½ cup Japanese soy sauce
1 cup mirin
1 tablespoon sugar

Chop chicken into ¼" cubes. Cut shallots into ½" lengths, using all the green part of the shallot. Alternately thread chicken and folded shallot pieces onto skewers. Set aside. Bring soy sauce, mirin and sugar to boil in a pot, stirring constantly, pour over skewered chicken and ensure that all chicken is coated. Drain sauce back into pot and boil again. Place chicken on hot grill or barbecue and turn frequently, brushing often with remaining sauce. Serve immediately.

DESSERTS

Tofu Yogurt   E W M

½ lb. soft tofu
1 large mango
½ lb. unsweetened crushed pineapple
3 teaspoons honey
vanilla essence (optional)

Beat tofu until fluffy, add mashed mango, pineapple and honey and mix well. Chill and serve.

Spiced Fruit Compote   E M W

½ lb. dried fruit w/out SO2 (pears, apricots, figs, apples etc.)
10 oz. apple juice
10 oz. water
1 cinnamon stick
2 whole cloves

Combine all ingredients in a pot and bring to boil. Simmer gently for 20 minutes. May be served hot or cold with Tofu Yogurt or Creamed Coconut Rice.

Creamed Coconut Rice   E W M

1 cup rice
3 cups coconut milk
½ cup apple juice
1 tablespoon honey

Boil rice in coconut milk until rice is tender and mixture is creamy. Add more coconut milk if necessary. Stir in honey and apple juice and serve hot or cold.

Tropical Rice Parfaits   E W M

2 cups Creamed Coconut Rice
2 bananas, sliced
2 passion fruit
1 mango, chopped, or 1 cup crushed pineapple

Fold fruit into rice and place in serving bowl. Decorate with strawberries or other fruit in season.

Spiced Oranges and Mango Cream   E W

6 oranges
1 tablespoon brown sugar
1 tablespoon honey
1 tablespoon lemon juice
½ teaspoon cinnamon

Peel oranges and separate carefully into segments, removing seeds and pit. Place in bowl and sprinkle with other ingredients. Toss until oranges are well coated, then marinate for 1 hour.

Cut some of the orange peel into very fine strips, drop into boiling water for 30 seconds, drain and rinse under cold water. Set aside.

Mango Cream

¼ lb. cream cheese, softened
½ lb. can mango slices, drained
1 cup whipped cream
1 tablespoon honey

Beat cream cheese until fluffy, add mango and beat until well blended. Mix in cream and honey and chill.

Place oranges in individual serving bowls. Spoon some Mango Cream onto each serving and garnish with orange peel shreds and a sprig of mint.

Soy Pancakes   W

2 eggs, separated
pinch salt
1 cup soy flour (may substitute brown rice flour)
1 cup skim milk
1 tablespoon raw sugar or honey

Beat egg yolks and milk. Stir in flour and salt. Beat egg whites until stiff, fold into mixture. Fry pancakes in a little butter. Serve with honey or fruit spread.

Brown Rice and Apple Pudding E W

1 cup brown rice
1½ cups unsweetened pure apple juice
½ cup water
1 cinnamon stick
pinch ground cloves
1 cup skim milk
¼ cup natural raisins
ground cinnamon

Apple Sauce
Peel and chop 5 medium apples and cook with 1 cup apple juice (extra).

Cook the rice with the apple juice, water, cinnamon stick and cloves, covered for about 40 minutes. Remove cinnamon stick and stir in milk and sultanas. Place apple sauce in a casserole dish and cover with rice mixture. Dust with cinnamon and bake in a moderate oven for 30 minutes.

CHAPTER 11

QUESTIONS AND ANSWERS

Q. I had a severe asthma attack after eating at a restaurant once, and I have been too afraid to eat out again. How can I know where it's safe to go to dinner?

A. The cause of your attack was probably a reaction to either metabisulfites or MSG, both of which are commonly present in restaurant food. Salads and seafood are commonly treated with sulfites to retain their fresh appearance. If you also drank wine, you may have increased the potential for a reaction even further, as wine often contains metabisulfite or sulfur dioxide. If MSG was the problem, you may be deficient in vitamin B6. This would increase your sensitivity to MSG. You should be taking the mineral molybdenum and vitamins B5, B12 and C to reduce your sensitivity to metabisulfites. An elimination diet would be in order to determine any food allergies. As far as knowing where it is safe to eat, you really need to speak to the management at the restaurant to know if their food contains the above additives.

Q. My mother says to give my children a daily dose of cod-liver oil for their asthma and frequent colds. Is this idea an old wife's tale or does it really work?

A. Cod liver or tuna oil is a good source of essential fatty acids, which are very important in reducing inflammation and strengthening immunity. It also contains considerable quantities of vitamin A, which is important for healthy mucous membranes and also immunity. Vitamin D, which is also present in fish oil, is very important in regulating hypersensitivity reactions. Follow your mother's advice if you want to improve asthma symptoms.

Q. **My husband has infrequent mild asthma. Whenever he eats anything containing vinegar or mustard, he coughs and complains of it 'taking his breath away'. Why is this happening?**

A. The reason for this kind of immediate reaction would be metabisulfite or sulfur dioxide in the vinegar based foods. Reduce sensitivity by taking molybdenum and vitamins B12, B5 and C. If salicylates are a problem supplement with glycine.

Q. **I recently began a detoxification program on the advice of a naturopath as I have had asthma and have been generally unwell for some time. I used to drink a lot of coffee and tea and often ate 'fast food.' After being on the program only a couple of days, my asthma began to worsen and become more frequent. What could be causing this?**

A. There are two major reasons for your problem. Your body would be releasing a lot of toxins which have been stored for some time and this can cause quite a number of reactions while your body is eliminating them. If you were a regular coffee drinker, your asthma might be worse as a result of your giving this up as coffee contains theophyllin—a drug that is commonly used as a bronchodilator in asthma.

Q. **My three year old daughter uses a nebulizer with Ventolin™ to keep her asthma under control. I am worried about the asthma, as it doesn't seem to be improving — it returns as soon as we stop using the medication, but I am also concerned about the Ventolin™ as it seems to 'hype her up' considerably. Could this be dangerous and could it have long-term effects?**

A. Yes, there are reports that Ventolin™ can be dangerous, especially with long-term use as this kind of drug dampens the normal cough reflex which is necessary to expel mucous. Ventolin™ works only on symptoms and does nothing to control the underlying inflammation of asthma. The cause of the asthma needs to be found and acted upon, and nutrients to reduce inflammation and strengthen immunity should be given. It is interesting to note that many nebulizer solutions contain preservatives and other additives, which can actually aggravate or precipitate asthma symptoms. Long-term use of Ventolin™ or the other sympathomimetics can reportedly be damaging to the heart.

Q. Can an ionizer be of benefit to asthmatics?

A. There is not a lot of scientific evidence to support the idea that ionizers are helpful.

Q. I am a forty-two year old male and for the past few months have noticed that I sometimes become tight in the chest and cough after drinking beer or wine. Could this be asthma, and does it mean that I will have to give up beer?

A. Yes, this does sound like asthma, and yes, you should really give up beer. Your problem could be metabisulfite sensitivity, in which case you would be helped by molybdenum and vitamins B5, B12 and C. The coldness of the drink could also cause bronchospasm. The other possibility is yeast sensitivity.

Q. My fifty year old mother worries me as she has asthma and yet refuses to give up smoking. She insists that a friend of hers who died of a severe asthma attack did so as a direct result of giving up smoking. How can I convince her that giving up will not induce a fatal attack?

A. If your mother has asthma, it will be the cigarettes and not the lack of them that will induce a fatal asthma attack. Smoking is ALWAYS contraindicated in asthma. What can happen, though, if someone who has been a heavy smoker gives up, a great deal of mucous can suddenly start to move out of the airways and this can cause problems if not expelled efficiently. Certain individuals can also become extremely sensitive to cigarette smoke after giving up smoking, having a severe reaction when exposed to smoke again.

Q. **Both of my preschool age children suffer from regular asthma attacks and both use a nebulizer. Our doctor feels the cause is probably pollens and dust, but after doing everything possible to eliminate these, the asthma is just as bad. After asking the doctor if any foods could be the problem, he said that it was extremely unlikely and dismissed the subject entirely. Should I pursue this further, and where do I begin?**

A. Yes, you should begin with an elimination diet. Keep a food/symptom diary and test for milk first of all. Consider metabisulfites and salicylates as other possible causes as these are very common causes of childhood asthma.

Q. **How important is it to remove perfumes and cosmetics, etc. from the house if a member of the family has asthma? I'm reluctant to throw them all out unless necessary.**

A. These products could definitely be a problem for anyone with asthma, especially if they are in the form of powders and sprays. Most perfumes contain benzene, toluene and xylene. All highly scented products and sprays should be avoided. It is possible to find less irritating products as substitutes for most cosmetics, etc. Or you can improve the body's detoxification system by taking supplements of glycine, taurine, vitamin B5, B1, B12, folic acid and vitamin B6

Q. **I suffered a severe asthma attack one night after eating Chinese food containing shrimp (I assumed this to be the cause at the time). I have eaten the same food once before though and nothing happened. Is it possible that the food was the problem?**

A. It is possible that a reaction to MSG was the cause of the attack as this is used extensively in most Chinese food. The other possibility is that you had an allergic reaction to the prawns or some other food, but if it were a true allergic reaction you probably would have had other symptoms as well, such as hives and facial swelling. The severity of a reaction to MSG is dependent on the amount ingested and on the level of vitamin B6 in the body. Vitamin B6 deficiency seems to be a major cause of MSG sensitivity.

Q. Our small country town seems to have a terribly high incidence of asthma, especially among the young children, and many of them are hospitalized regularly. I have often wondered about the wheat and corn which are the major crops farmed here, as being possible contributing factors. Also, many of the farmers use aerial spraying of fertilizers and pesticides. The climate is hot, dry and dusty. Are these likely causes of the problem?

A. It is not surprising that there is such a high incidence of asthma in your area. Wheat dust, pesticide spray and dry, dusty air are all major triggers of asthma. It is likely that the children there are having a problem with their immune systems right from the start. The constant bombardment from all of these substances in the air is not giving anyone's health much of a chance. It is essential that the mineral molybdenum and vitamin C, taurine, B5 and B12 be given to counteract the toxic effects of chemical exposure. Homoeopathic remedies can often be effective in eliminating toxins from the body. The children should be checked for wheat sensitivity, as well as for other foods and inhaled allergens. An elimination diet should be followed. Immunity should be boosted and inflammation reduced with the correct nutritional supplements. Essential fatty acid supplements, cabbage, garlic and onions should be consumed regularly. A static-type air filter should be used in the home, and on days when aerial spraying is taking place, stay indoors with windows closed. If the air is very dry, it would be worthwhile having a humidifier, as dry air is very irritating to airways. Outdoor activities should also be avoided on windy days to reduce exposure to wheat dust and pollens. Reduce exposure to all chemicals in the form of food additives and household products such as sprays, etc.

Q My three-year old suffers from asthma (mainly at night) and has quite a lot of mucous with this. We have bought a vaporizer but I'm not sure that it is helping at all. Are vaporizers beneficial in any way?

A. Vaporizers help to make mucous less sticky and thick so that it can be more easily expelled. Various substances such as eucalyptus, menthol or camphor, which are often used with the vaporizer, can all help to clear congestion as well.

Q. **Our four year old son has 'enlarged' tonsils and they frequently become inflamed. Recently he started to cough a lot, mainly at night, and the doctor tells me that the cause is asthma. He has prescribed Bricanyl. I feel skeptical about the medication as well as the diagnosis. How do I know it's really asthma? Couldn't the cough be simply related to his tonsil problem?**

A. This might not be asthma. The only way to be sure of this diagnosis is by measuring peak flow to determine fluctuations in respiratory function. Simply using a peak flow meter at home can do this. It sounds as though this child's adenoids should be checked. Immune boosting and anti-inflammatory nutrients should be taken. Bioflavonoids may help to reduce swelling and inflammation of the tonsils.

Q. **How successful are desensitization injections? My doctor has suggested I try them as I am strongly allergic to a number of substances. Could they be dangerous?**

A. Desensitization or allergy immunotherapy works for some people, but only for certain allergens. The course of treatment is usually quite long, and of course, there is no guarantee that it will 'cure' your allergy permanently. There is risk of a severe reaction occurring in very sensitive individuals.

Q. **My mother is always telling me that my asthma is caused by my being such a 'nervous' person and that I 'worry myself into an attack'. The idea that my asthma has a neurotic basis upsets me. Could it really be all in my mind?**

A. Anxiety or emotional upsets are very common triggers of asthma in a large number of people. It is possible that emotional factors could play a large part in your asthma, but this does not mean that your symptoms are 'all in your mind'—they are in fact very real and should always be taken seriously. Relaxation therapy is extremely helpful for many asthma sufferers.

Q. **Is tartrazine really as dangerous as all the recent publicity claims? It seems to be in a great many foods that my children love to eat (both of whom have chronic, mild asthma).**

A. Tartrazine™ (artificial coloring agent) has the potential to cause a variety of adverse effects in sensitive individuals. Some of the effects, which have been widely reported, include: asthma, skin rashes, urticaria and hyperactivity. Its use has been banned in several countries in Europe, but it is still to be found in an amazing range of foods here in the U.S. Tartrazine also increases excretion of zinc from the body. Zinc is extremely important for the functioning of the immune system. It is also important for the activation of vitamin B6, a common vitamin deficiency in asthmatics.

Q. **A lady I know swears by vitamin B6 as a remedy for asthma attacks. She says that by taking some when she feels an attack coming on, she is able to stop the symptoms occurring. How can this be possible? I didn't think that vitamins could be used in this way.**

A. Some people seem to have a problem metabolizing vitamin B6 and therefore require larger quantities than others. This problem can obviously lead to a deficiency, which often seems to be a factor in asthma. B6 helps to reduce inflammation. Many people with asthma have had beneficial results with B6 supplements. Or better still, supplement with the active form of B6, pyridoxal-5-phosphate.

Q. **My toddler's asthma improved greatly when he was placed on a milk-free diet, but the problem is, he won't drink soy milk and I am concerned about the nutrients he is missing. What should I do?**

A. The nutrients you should be most concerned about are calcium, protein and vitamins A and D. Salmon and tuna (oil-packed) are excellent sources of all these nutrients.

Drinks can be made using cashew milk, coconut milk and a wide variety of fruit juices. Calcium is also found in legumes, dark green vegetables and sesame seeds. Cod liver oil contains large amounts of vitamins A and D as well as essential fatty acids that are very important for immunity. As with any restricted diet, supplements should be taken, especially if the child is a fussy eater.

Q. What are the best vitamin supplements to reduce the severity of asthma?

A. It is essential that asthma patients supplement their diet with vitamins and minerals. Supplements may reduce inflammation, improve digestion, support liver detoxification, regulate cellular energetics and oxygenation and improve mental outlook. Vitamin B6, zinc, B12, folate, magnesium, quercetin, vitamins C & E would be best supplements to take. Fish oil intake (tuna, cod liver oil and/or evening primrose oil) should be part of the diet. If chemical sensitivity is a problem, detoxifying nutrients such as taurine, glycine, B5, B1, choline and methionine should be added to the above list.

To improve general energy, Lipoic Acid and Co Enzyme Q10 may be of some assistance.

Q. If I have an acute mild asthma attack, what should I do?

A. Drink Black coffee. It contains theophylline, which causes bronchial relaxation. Vitamin C (2 gms.) Calcium (400 mg.) and Vitamin D (400 i.u.), Co Enzyme Q10 (200 mg.) supplement can reduce the severity of the asthma attack within the hour. However, if the attack is severe, you need to treat it with medication. Discuss this issue with your doctor.

Q. What dosage range should I use for my children when I am supplementing with vitamins and minerals?

A. As a general rule of thumb, children under the age of 10 use ⅕ to ⅓ the adult range that has been recommended throughout the book. The younger the child, the smaller the dose.

CHAPTER 12

COMMON MYTHS AND MISCONCEPTIONS ABOUT ASTHMA

1. **'Children will usually grow out of asthma, so there's no need to worry too much about treatment unless an attack is severe.'**

Research has shown that if asthma isn't controlled, even when seemingly very mild, it will often worsen and have serious long-term effects on health. It is true that many children become completely symptom-free as they grow up, but this is only likely to happen if their condition has been managed adequately during early childhood. Sometimes asthma seems to disappear only to return again a few years later. This is why every effort must be made to overcome asthma as soon as it occurs—by using the appropriate treatment, avoiding trigger factors and improving general health and immunity. Parents should never wait for their children to 'grow out of asthma'.

2. **'It can't be asthma as there is no wheeze.'**

Many people still think of asthma as an audible wheeze with or without other symptoms. The truth is, asthma does not affect everyone in the same way, and in many cases there is no obvious wheezing to be heard. Many people who suffer from bouts of chest tightness, coughing or shortness of breath on exertion, for example, may actually be suffering from asthma and not know it. Doctors are now recognizing more and more cases of what they refer to as **'atypical asthma'**. A classic example of atypical asthma is shortness of breath with no other obvious symptoms at all. Diagnosis is usually confirmed when an improvement in lung function can be brought about with the use of an inhaled bronchodilator (lung function is measured using peak flow or spirometry). And what exactly is a wheeze? A wheeze is generally defined as a coarse, whistling sound which is produced when partial obstruction of airflow in the lungs occurs. It is not always present in airway obstruction, and it will usually not be heard if the breathing is very shallow.

3. 'Asthma occurs only in attacks.'

Although sudden, acute attacks of asthma with periods of remission in between are quite common, many people have a slow, insidious deterioration in lung function which may span over weeks or months. It is possible for people to have chronic (long-term), mild asthma and not be aware of it for some time.

The primary feature of asthma—inflammation—may be present for varying lengths of time without causing terribly severe, acute symptoms. Regular health checks are important, and any vague, chronic symptoms such as unexplained fatigue or shortness of breath should be thoroughly investigated. Many people suffer from what would be better described as 'bouts' of asthma, where they might have a mild wheeze and cough for a week or so, with this happening perhaps only a couple of times a year. This is common with people who develop asthma after having a cold, for example. Children, especially, will often suffer from a couple of bouts during winter and then will be fine throughout the rest of the year.

4. 'Babies under twelve months of age don't get asthma.'

Asthma is not common under the age of one year but it certainly can and does occur. The distinguishing feature is the recurring nature of asthma symptoms. Many babies develop problems such as bronchitis or croup which may cause a severe cough, but these tend to be one-off episodes which usually do not recur. Accurate diagnosis is very important, but is often difficult as babies frequently have a persistent cough as the only symptom of asthma.

5. 'People with asthma shouldn't play sports or do anything strenuous.'

Not every person with asthma develops symptoms as a result of exercise. Even though many people do have exercise-induced asthma, it certainly does not mean that they cannot or should not exercise (one in ten athletes on the Australian Olympic team has asthma). It is actually of vital importance as part of their treatment for all people with asthma to keep fit by adopting an appropriate exercise program. Activities and sports which involve brief intervals rather than sustained endurance are usually recommended, but, whatever the type of exercise, it is important that it is regular. People with asthma are usually advised against scuba diving.

6. 'Ignore it and it will go away.'

This is an extremely foolish attitude and one which has probably led to many tragedies. The facts are loud and clear — putting off treatment in the hope that asthma will simply disappear is dangerous. Asthma is sometimes ignored by people who feel inadequate because of their condition. They may (wrongly) feel it reflects a weakness not only in their body, but in their mind. People who believe their asthma is 'all in their mind' may try to rely on willpower alone to control symptoms. Emotion may be a major trigger factor in some cases, but a severe asthma attack requires prompt medical attention regardless of the cause. Asthma must not be ignored.

7. 'Asthma is merely contractions in the muscles of the airways and all you need to do is stop the contractions with a drug such as Ventolin™.'

Even doctors believed up until recently that this muscle contraction (bronchospasm) was the hallmark of asthma. They now know that the primary feature is inflammation and that this needs to be controlled if the bronchospasm is to be controlled effectively in the long-term. Because of this knowledge, treatment has changed somewhat in recent years to a much more widespread use of preventive and anti-inflammatory drugs such as Becotide™ or Intal™, and less reliance on bronchodilators alone, such as Ventolin™. The underlying inflammation in chronic asthma causes the airways to be more sensitive to various triggers, so it is obvious that this needs to be treated. It is now recognized that the long-term, frequent use of bronchodilators (which provide symptomatic relief only) without any other treatment or preventive measures can actually be dangerous.

8. **'It's not really asthma—there's no history of asthma in our family, and anyway, asthma is just a fashionable disease at the moment.'**

Unfortunately, a number of people will vehemently reject a diagnosis of asthma because of misunderstanding and fear. Some parents of young children in particular, are often reluctant to accept such a diagnosis, and will sometimes flatly refuse to believe the doctor. If you're really doubtful, it doesn't hurt to get a second opinion. However, there is certainly no disputing the fact that the incidence of asthma has risen in recent years. Also, it is possible to have asthma in the absence of a family history of the condition, although it is much more common in those inherently predisposed.

9. **'Asthma is always a gravely serious disease which severely affects the lifestyle of sufferers.'**

This misconception has led to a great deal of anxiety—and in some cases, denial of the diagnosis. In the **majority** of cases, asthma never reaches the point where it is life-threatening or causing any great disturbance to lifestyle.

What many people don't seem to realize, is that asthma can be very mild and is frequently little more than an inconvenience. Of course, anyone who has ever suffered from asthma should be prepared and know exactly what to do in the case of an emergency, but most people are able to enjoy a full, normal life with very few adjustments or restrictions. After all, asthma is really just a word for a group of symptoms which can vary enormously in severity, but which are **usually** mild if the condition is treated properly.

OVERCOMING ASTHMA:
SUMMARY OF MAJOR POINTS

◆ Identify dietary or environmental allergens and take steps to avoid them. Use elimination diet if necessary.

◆ Reduce exposure to dust, mold, pollens and other common irritants. Follow guidelines in Chapter 6—Practical Help.

◆ Don't smoke, avoid exposure to other people's cigarette smoke and avoid other forms of pollution as much as possible.

◆ Reduce exposure to chemicals. Stop using aerosol sprays and other irritant products.

◆ Take steps to avoid asthma triggers associated with your occupation.

◆ Learn to breathe through the nose—not the mouth.

◆ Practice breathing and relaxation exercises daily.

◆ Take some form of regular (daily if possible) exercise. This should not be too strenuous if you are not used to it— walking or swimming is ideal.

◆ Take steps to reduce stress.

◆ Eat only natural, unprocessed foods. Avoid additives.

◆ Ensure optimal nutritional intake. Supplement with immune-boosting, detoxifying and anti-inflammatory nutrients.

◆ Ensure adequate fluid intake. Drink 2–3 quarts of pure water per day.

◆ Treat any colds or rhinitis promptly. See Chapter 8.

◆ Improve digestion.

GUIDELINES FOR HEALTHY EATING
AND BENEFICIAL DIGESTION

- Avoid refined and processed foods, especially white flour and sugar and foods made with these e.g. cakes, biscuits, etc. Bake your own using whole grain flour.
- Avoid foods which contain chemical additives and pollutants.
- Ensure that your diet contains a wide VARIETY of HIGH QUALITY foods which include: whole grain cereals and breads, lean meat, fish and poultry, nuts, beans and seeds and plenty of fresh fruits and vegetables.
- Drink at least 2–3 quarts of fluid every day. Include plenty of plain water (spring or filtered is best), fresh fruit or vegetable juices, herb teas. Avoid or restrict tea, coffee and cocoa.
- Restrict salt, sugar and alcohol intake.
- Include plenty of fiber in your diet with whole grains and raw fruits and vegetables.
- Eat regularly. Five or six small meals per day are preferable to 3 large ones.
- Don't overcook food, especially vegetables and fruit. Steam lightly, using a minimum of water.
- To retain essential fatty acids in the diet, use only olive oil or butter for cooking, and use cold-pressed safflower or sunflower oils for salads. Avoid polyunsaturated oils which have been hydrogenated, including margarine.
- Eat cold water varieties of fish three times per week (cod, tuna, and herring).
- Increase consumption of garlic, onion, ginger and chilies.

FOR BENEFICIAL DIGESTION:

- Eat slowly and chew food well. Don't overeat.
- Avoid fried and fatty foods.
- Don't go to bed with a full stomach—the last meal of the day should be light, and should be eaten 3 to 4 hours before going to bed.
- Supplement with digestive enzymes if necessary.
- If indigestion or heartburn is a problem—follow the above guidelines, check for food sensitivities, elevate the

head of the bed by at least 6 inches, and increase intake of vitamin A, silicon and magnesium. Foods which commonly cause heartburn in sensitive individuals include: chocolate, alcohol, citrus fruits, tomato products, coffee, and salicylate-rich foods. Don't smoke, as this can lower esophageal sphincter pressure and aggravate or cause heartburn.

If not sensitive to salicylate, take two teaspoon of apple cider vinegar in water with meals.

NUTRIENT SUPPLEMENT OPTIONS

For **mild acute attacks of asthma** the following should be taken:

Black coffee (no sugar or milk)—contains the drug theophylline—1 cup.

Pyridoxine-5-phosphate	10 mg.
Quercetin	600 mg.
Co Enzyme Q10	100 mg.
Calcium	400 mg.
Vitamin D	100 i.u.

Nutritional Supplement Options

Multi-vitamin capsule should be taken by every asthmatic

Tuna Oil	3 tsp./ day	(Rich in omega 3 fatty acids)
Pyridoxal-5-Phosphate	10 mgs. x 3 per day	(Activated vitamin B6)
Vitamin C as		
Ca & Mg salts of vitamin C	2 gm./day	(Improve immunity)
Zinc (as sulfate)	20 mg./day	(Activates Vitamin B6 improves immunity)
Vitamin B12	300–900 mg./day	(Detoxifying nutrient)
Folic Acid	400–900 mg./day	(Detoxifying nutrient)
Quercetin	600–1000 mg./day	(Anti-inflammatory, anti-viral, inhibits PAF)
Alpha Tocopherol		
(Vitamin E)	600 mg./day	(antioxidant, immune stimulant)
Gamma Tocopherol	50–100 mg.	(antioxidant, quenches the peroxynitrite ion)

CoEnzyme Q10	90–180 mg./day	(Improves cellular energetics, prevents anaphylactic reactions)
Taurine	1000–2000 mg./day	(Improves chemical detoxification)
Magnesium (as ascorbate/orotate)	0–400 mg./day	(Muscle relaxant, improve cellular function)
Tyrosine	400–1000 mg./day	(Improve adrenal exhaustion)
Lipoic Acid	50–100 mg./day	(antioxidant, reduces inflammation)
Pancreatin (Enzyme)	1 Capsule with meal	(improves digestion)
Ginkgo biloba extract	160 mg.	(regulates platelet activating factor)
Ginger extract	375 mg.	(modulates thromboxane synthesis)

N.B. All supplementary dosages refer to adults. Infant and children require lower dosages. Refer to your Physician for advice.

REFERENCES AND FURTHER READING

CHAPTER 1

1: Kumar RK. Bronchial asthma: recent advances. *Indian J Pediatr.* 2000 Apr;67(4):293–8. Review.

2: Lemanske RF Jr. Inflammatory events in asthma: an expanding equation. *J Allergy Clin Immunol.* 2000 Jun;105(6 Pt 2):S633–6. Review.

3: Law KW, Ng KK, Yuen KN, Ho CS. Detecting asthma and bronchial hyperresponsiveness in children. *Hong Kong Med J.* 2000 Mar;6(1):99–104. Review.

4: Gern JE. Viral and bacterial infections in the development and progression of asthma. *J Allergy Clin Immunol.* 2000 Feb;105(2 Pt 2):S497–502. Review.

5: Banks DE, Tarlo SM. Important issues in occupational asthma. *Curr Opin Pulm Med.* 2000 Jan;6(1):37–42. Review.

6: Pekkanen J, Pearce N. Defining asthma in epidemiological studies. *Eur Respir J.* 1999 Oct;14(4):951–7. Review.

7: Miralles-Lopez J, Guillen-Grima F et al Bronchial asthma prevalence in childhood. *Allergol Immunopathol* (Madr). 1999 Jul–Aug;27(4):200–11. Review.

8: Weiss ST. Gene by environment interaction and asthma. *Clin Exp Allergy.* 1999 Jun;29 Suppl 2:96–9. Review.

9: Busse WW, Banks-Schlegel S, Wenzel SE. Pathophysiology of severe asthma. *J Allergy Clin Immunol.* 2000 Dec;106(6):1033–42.

10: Janahi IA, Elidemir O et al. Recurrent milk aspiration produces changes in airway mechanics, lung eosinophilia, and goblet cell hyperplasia in a murine model. *Pediatr Res.* 2000 Dec;48(6):776–81.

11: Tarlo SM, Leung K et al. Asthmatic subjects symptomatically worse at work : prevalence and characterization among a general asthma clinic population. *Chest.* 2000 Nov;118(5):1309–14.

12: Leynaert B, Neukirch F et al. Epidemiologic evidence for asthma and rhinitis comorbidity. *J Allergy Clin Immunol.* 2000 Nov;106(5 Pt 2):201–205.

13: Reinisch F, Harrison RJ et al. Physician reports of work-related asthma in california, 1993–1996. *Am J Ind Med.* 2001 Jan;39(1):72–83.

14: Tan KS, Thomson NC. Asthma in pregnancy. *Am J Med.* 2000 Dec 15;109(9):727–33

15: Doyle LW, Cheung MM et al. Birth weight <1501 g and respiratory health at age 14. *Arch Dis Child.* 2001 Jan;84(1):40–44.

16: Ramadour M, Burel C et al. Prevalence of asthma and rhinitis in relation to long-term exposure to gaseousair pollutants. *Allergy.* 2000 Dec;55(12):1163–9.

CHAPTER 2

1: Carr MJ, Hunter DD, Undem BJ. Neurotrophins and asthma. *Curr Opin Pulm Med.* 2001 Jan;7(1):1–7.

2: Rylander R, Lin R. (1—>3)-beta-D-glucan—relationship to indoor air-related symptoms, allergy and asthma. *Toxicology.* 2000 Nov 2;152(1-3):47–52.

3: Lapa e Silva JR et al. Endotoxins, asthma, and allergic immune responses. *Toxicology.* 2000 Nov 2;152(1-3):31–5.

4: Droste JH, Wieringa MH, Weyler JJ et al. Does the use of antibiotics in early childhood increase the risk of asthma and allergic disease? *Clin Exp Allergy.* 2000 Nov;30(11):1548–53.

5: Kraneveld AD, James DE et al. Excitatory non-adrenergic-non-cholinergic neuropeptides: key players in asthma. *Eur J Pharmacol.* 2000 Sep 29;405(1-3):113–29.

6: von Hertzen LC. Puzzling associations between childhood infections and the later occurrence of asthma and atopy. *Ann Med.* 2000 Sep;32(6):397–400.

7: Leff AR. Role of leukotrienes in bronchial hyperresponsiveness and cellular responses in airways. *Thorax.* 2000 Oct;55 Suppl 2:S32–7. Review

8: Brightling CE, Ward R et al. Induced sputum inflammatory mediator concentrations in eosinophilic bronchitis and asthma. *Am J Respir Crit Care Med.* 2000 Sep;162(3 Pt 1):878–82.

9: Li JT, Sheeler RD et al. Consultation for asthma: results of a generalist survey. *Ann Allergy Asthma Immunol.* 1999 Sep;83(3):203–6.

10: Wenzel SE, Schwartz LB et al. Evidence that severe asthma can be divided pathologically into two inflammatory subtypes with distinct physiologic and clinical characteristics. *Am J Respir Crit Care Med.* 1999 Sep;160(3):1001–8.

11: Henriksen AH, Sue-Chu M et al. Exhaled and nasal NO levels in allergic rhinitis: relation to sensitization, pollen season and bronchial hyperresponsiveness. *Eur Respir J.* 1999 Feb;13(2):301–6.

12: Varney VA, Holgate ST. Allergy testing in respiratory medicine. *Br J Hosp Med.* 1996 Oct 16-Nov 5;56(8):406–8. Review.

13: Martinez FD, Wright AL et al. Asthma and wheezing in the first six years of life. The Group Health Medical Associates. *N Engl J Med.* 1995 Jan 19;332(3):133–8.

14: Ahlstedt S, Peterson CG, Enander I. Update in allergy testing in childhood asthma: how do you know whether you are successfully controlling the patient's inflammation? *Pediatr Pulmonol Suppl.* 1995;11:32–3.

15: Salkie ML. Role of clinical laboratory in allergy testing. *Clin Biochem.* 1994 Oct;27(5):343–55. Review.

16: Mojsoski N. [Bronchial asthma and methemoglobinemia caused by milk allergy]. *Plucne Bolesti*. 1991 Jan-Jun;43(1-2):83–5).

17: Dhungat AJ, Desai SA et al. Immunoglobulins and allergy mediators in bronchial asthma. *J Assoc Physicians India*. 1990 Aug;38(8):542–4.

18: Sethi S, Sarkar B, Gupta SR. A study of intradermal allergy testing in bronchial asthma. *Indian J Chest Dis Allied Sci*. 1986 Jul-Sep;28(3):105–8.

19: Baker JC, Duncanson RC et al. Development of a standardized methodology for double-blind, placebo-controlled food challenge in patients with brittle asthma and perceived food intolerance. *J Am Diet Assoc*. 2000 Nov;100(11):1361–7.

20: Tariq SM, Matthews SM et al. Egg allergy in infancy predicts respiratory allergic disease by 4 years of age. *Pediatr Allergy Immunol*. 2000 Aug;11(3):162–7.

21: Wuthrich B. Lethal or life-threatening allergic reactions to food. *J Investig Allergol Clin Immunol*. 2000 Mar-Apr;10(2):59–65. Review.

22: Musmand JJ, Daul CB, Lehrer SB. Crustacea allergy. *Clin Exp Allergy*. 1993 Sep;23(9):722-32. Review.

23: Vally H, de Klerk N, Thompson PJ. Alcoholic drinks: important triggers for asthma. *J Allergy Clin Immunol*. 2000 Mar;105(3):462–7.

24: Vally H, de Klerk N, Thompson PJ. Asthma induced by alcoholic drinks: a new food allergy questionnaire. *Aust N Z J Public Health*. 1999 Dec;23(6):590–4.

25: Tasman AJ, Witzel A et al. [The skin prick test and nasal provocation test with individually prepared flour extracts in patients with bakers' rhinitis and asthma]. *HNO*. 1999 Aug;47(8):718–22.

26: Woessner KM, Simon RA, Stevenson DD. Monosodium glutamate sensitivity in asthma. *J Allergy Clin Immunol*. 1999 Aug;104(2 Pt 1):305–10.

27: Rance F, Kanny G et al. Food hypersensitivity in children: clinical aspects and distribution of allergens. *Pediatr Allergy Immunol*. 1999 Feb;10(1):33–8.

28: Curioni A, Santucci B et al. Urticaria from beer: an immediate hypersensitivity reaction due to a 10-kDa protein derived from barley. *Clin Exp Allergy*. 1999 Mar;29(3):407–13.

29: Arai Y, Muto H, Sano Y, Ito K. [Food and food additives hypersensitivity in adult asthmatics. III. Adverse reaction to sulfites in adult asthmatics]. *Arerugi*. 1998 Nov;47(11):1163–7. PMID: 9893332; UI: 99109210

30: Vally H, Carr A et al. Wine-induced asthma: a placebo-controlled assessment of its pathogenesis. *J Allergy Clin Immunol*. 1999 Jan;103(1 Pt 1):41–6.

31: Casas R, Djerf P et al. Circulating cat allergen and immune complexes in cat-allergic children. *Clin Exp Allergy*. 1998 Oct;28(10):1258–63.

32: Bergmann R, Woodcock A. Whole population or high-risk group? Childhood asthma. *Eur Respir J Suppl*. 1998 Jul;27:9s–12s. Review.

33: Zhong NS. New insights into risk factors of asthma. *Respirology*. 1996 Sep;1(3):159–66. Review.

34: Song CH. Skin sensitization in asthmatic children less than 36 months of age. *Ann Allergy Asthma Immunol*. 1997 Sep;79(3):273–6.

35: Huss K, Adkinson NF Jr et al. House dust mite and cockroach exposure are strong risk factors for positive allergy skin test responses in the Childhood Asthma Management Program. *J Allergy Clin Immunol*. 2001 Jan;107(1):48–54.

36: Litonjua AA, Carey VJ et al. Exposure to cockroach allergen in the home is associated with incident doctor-diagnosed asthma and recurrent wheezing. *J Allergy Clin Immunol*. 2001 Jan;107(1):41–47.

37: Li JT, Andrist D et al. Accuracy of patient prediction of allergy skin test results. *Ann Allergy Asthma Immunol*. 2000 Nov;85(5):382–4.

38: Nagakura T, Matsuda S et al. Dietary supplementation with fish oil rich in omega-3 polyunsaturated fatty acids in children with bronchial asthma. *Eur Respir J*. 2000 Nov;16(5):861–5.

39: [No authors listed]. Aspirin intolerance and related syndromes: a multidisciplinary approach. Proceedings of an international symposium. Rome, 11–13 November 1999. *Thorax*. 2000 Oct;55 Suppl 2:S1–90.

40: Hartert TV, Dworski RT et al. Prostaglandin E(2) decreases allergen-stimulated release of prostaglandin D(2) in airways of subjects with asthma. *Am J Respir Crit Care Med*. 2000 Aug;162(2 Pt 1):637–40.

41: Bisgaard H. Role of leukotrienes in asthma pathophysiology. *Pediatr Pulmonol*. 2000 Aug;30(2):166–76. Review.

42: Hassig A, Liang WX, Stampfli K. Bronchial asthma: information on phytotherapy with essential fatty acids. Interactions between essential fatty acids and steroid hormones. *Med Hypotheses*. 2000 Jan;54(1):72–4.

43: Horrocks LA, Yeo YK. Health benefits of docosahexaenoic acid. *Pharmacol Res*. 1999 Sep;40(3):211–25. Review.

44: Weiland SK, von Mutius E et al. Intake of trans fatty acids and prevalence of childhood asthma and allergies in Europe. ISAAC Steering Committee. *Lancet*. 1999 Jun 12;353(9169):2040–1. .

45: Villani F, Comazzi R et al. Effect of dietary supplementation with polyunsaturated fatty acids on bronchial hyperreactivity in subjects with seasonal asthma. *Respiration*. 1998;65(4):265–9.

46: Hodge L, Salome CM et al. Effect of dietary intake of omega-3 and omega-6 fatty acids on severity of asthma in children. *Eur Respir J*. 1998 Feb;11(2):361–5.

47: Broughton KS, Johnson CS et al. Reduced asthma symptoms with n-3 fatty acid ingestion are related to 5-series leukotriene production. *Am J Clin Nutr*. 1997 Apr;65(4):1011–7.

48: Masuev KA. [The effect of polyunsaturated fatty acids on the biochemical indices of bronchial asthma patients]. *Ter Arkh*. 1997;69(3):33–5.

49: Jones PD, Gibson PG, Henry RL. The prevalence of asthma appears to be inversely related to the incidence of typhoid and tuberculosis: hypothesis to explain the variation in asthma prevalence around the world. *Med Hypotheses.* 2000 Jul;55(1):40–2.

50: Marshall GD Jr, Agarwal SK. Stress, immune regulation, and immunity: applications for asthma. *Allergy Asthma Proc.* 2000 Jul–Aug;21(4):241–6.

51: Liu AH.Allergy and asthma: classic TH2 diseases. *Allergy Asthma Proc.* 2000 Jul–Aug;21(4):227–30.

52: Bjorksten B. Environment and infant immunity. *Proc Nutr Soc.* 1999 Aug;58(3):729–32. Review.

53: Palma-Carlos AG, Palma-Carlos ML et al. Immunological control of immunotherapy in asthma. *Allerg Immunol* (Paris). 1986 Apr;18(4):21–6. Review.

54: Kaad PH, Ostergaard PA. The hazard of mould hyposensitization in children with asthma. *Clin Allergy.* 1982 May;12(3):317-20.

CHAPTER 3

1: Lipworth BJ. The comparative safety/efficacy ratio of HFA-BDP. *Respir Med.* 2000 Sep;94 Suppl D:S21–6. Review.

2: Donohue JF. The expanding role of long-acting beta-agonists. *Chest.* 2000 Aug;118(2):28–5. Review.

3: Barnes PJ. New directions in allergic diseases: mechanism-based anti-inflammatory therapies. *J Allergy Clin Immunol.* 2000 Jul;106(1 Pt 1):5–16. Review.

4: Thien F. Leukotriene antagonists. Do they offer new hope for asthmatics? *Aust Fam Physician.* 2000 Jun;29(6):547-51. Review.

5: Gonda I. The ascent of pulmonary drug delivery. *J Pharm Sci.* 2000 Jul;89(7):940–5. Review.

6: Bjorksten B. Unmet needs in the treatment of asthmatic children and adolescents: 2. *Clin Exp Allergy.* 2000 Jun;30 Suppl 1:73–6. Review.

7: Gupta G. Anti-leukotrienes in asthma: yet to arrive. *Indian J Pediatr.* 2000 Feb;67(2):113–7. Review.

8: Fick RB Jr. Anti-IgE as novel therapy for the treatment of asthma. *Curr Opin Pulm Med.* 1999 Jan;5(1):76–80. Review.

9: Wood-Baker R, Walters EH. Corticosteroids for acute exacerbations of chronic obstructive pulmonary disease. *Cochrane Database Syst Rev.* 2000;(2):CD001288. Review.

10: Wilson AJ, Gibson PG, Coughlan J. Long acting beta-agonists versus theophylline for maintenance treatment of asthma. *Cochrane Database Syst Rev.* 2000;(2):CD001281. Review.

11: Everard ML, Bara A, Kurian M. Anti-cholinergic drugs for wheeze in children under the age of two years. *Cochrane Database Syst Rev.* 2000;(2):CD001279. Review.

12: Appleton S, Smith B, Veale A, Bara A. Long-acting beta2-agonists for chronic obstructive pulmonary disease. *Cochrane Database Syst Rev.* 2000;(2):CD001104. Review.

13: Kercsmar CM. Aerosol treatment of acute asthma: and the winner is... *J Pediatr.* 2000 Apr;136(4):428–31. Review.

14: Giembycz MA. Phosphodiesterase 4 inhibitors and the treatment of asthma: where are we now and where do we go from here? *Drugs.* 2000 Feb;59(2):193–212. Review.

15: [No authors listed]. Salmeterol/fluticasone propionate combination product in asthma. An evaluation of its cost effectiveness vs fluticasone propionate. *Pharmacoeconomics.* 1999;16 Suppl 2:i-viii, 1–34. Review.

16: Lim TK. Asthma management: evidence based studies and their implications for cost-efficacy. *Asian Pac J Allergy Immunol.* 1999 Sep;17(3):195–202. Review.

17: Hannemann LA. What is new in asthma: new dry powder inhalers. *J Pediatr Health Care.* 1999 Jul–Aug;13(4):159–65. Review.

18: Nelson HS. Allergen and irritant control: importance and implementation. *Clin Cornerstone.* 1998 Aug–Sep;1(2):57–68. Review.

19: Konig P. The effects of cromolyn sodium and nedocromil sodium in early asthma prevention. *J Allergy Clin Immunol.* 2000 Feb;105(2 Pt 2):S575–81. Review.

20: Volsko T, Reed MD. Drugs used in the treatment of asthma: a review of clinical pharmacology and aerosol drug delivery. *Respir Care Clin N Am.* 2000 Mar;6(1):41–55. Review.

CHAPTER 4

1: Dworski R. Oxidant stress in asthma. *Thorax.* 2000 Oct;55 Suppl 2:S51–3. Review.

2: Jones AP. Asthma and the home environment. *J Asthma.* 2000 Apr;37(2):103–24. Review.

3: Mudway IS, Kelly FJ. Ozone and the lung: a sensitive issue. *Mol Aspects Med.* 2000 Feb–Apr;21(1–2):1–48. Review.

4: Bauer V, Bauer F. Reactive oxygen species as mediators of tissue protection and injury. *Gen Physiol Biophys.* 1999 Oct;18 Spec No:7–14. Review.

5: Blomberg A. Airway inflammatory and antioxidant responses to oxidative and particulate air pollutants—experimental exposure studies in humans. *Clin Exp Allergy.* 2000 Mar;30(3):310–7. Review.

6: Casillas AM, Hiura T, Li N, Nel AE. Enhancement of allergic inflammation by diesel exhaust particles: permissive role of reactive oxygen species. *Ann Allergy Asthma Immunol.* 1999 Dec;83(6 Pt 2):624–9. Review.

7: Fogarty A, Britton J. Nutritional issues and asthma. *Curr Opin Pulm Med.* 2000 Jan;6(1):86–9. Review.

8: Greene LS. Asthma, oxidant stress, and diet. *Nutrition.* 1999 Nov-Dec;15(11–12):899–907. Review.

9: Morcillo EJ, Estrela J, Cortijo J. Oxidative stress and pulmonary inflammation: pharmacological intervention with antioxidants. *Pharmacol Res.* 1999 Nov;40(5):393–404. Review.

10: Smit HA, Grievink L, Tabak C. Dietary influences on chronic obstructive lung disease and asthma: a review of the epidemiological evidence. *Proc Nutr Soc.* 1999 May;58(2):309–19. Review.

11: Horrocks LA, Yeo YK. Health benefits of docosahexaenoic acid. *Pharmacol Res.* 1999 Sep;40(3):211–25. Review.

12: Woods RK, Thien FC, Abramson MJ. Dietary marine fatty acids (fish oil) for asthma. *Cochrane Database Syst Rev.* 2000;(2):CD001283. Review.

13: Schwartz J. Role of polyunsaturated fatty acids in lung disease. *Am J Clin Nutr.* 2000 Jan;71(1 Suppl):393S–6S. Review.

14: Goldstein MF, Fallon JJ Jr, Harning R. Chronic glucocorticoid therapy-induced osteoporosis in patients with obstructive lung disease. *Chest.* 1999 Dec;116(6):1733–49. Review.

15: Saris NE, Mervaala E, Karppanen H, Khawaja JA, Lewenstam A. Magnesium. An update on physiological, clinical and analytical aspects. *Clin Chim Acta.* 2000 Apr;294(1–2):1–26. Review.

16: Swain R, Kaplan-Machlis B. Magnesium for the next millennium. *South Med J.* 1999 Nov;92(11):1040–7. Review.

17: Alberts WM. Divalent cations and bronchodilation in asthma. *Crit Care Med.* 1999 Jun;27(6):1056–7. Review.

18: Dib JG, Engstrom FM, Sisca TS, Tiu RM. Intravenous magnesium sulfate treatment in a child with status asthmaticus. *Am J Health Syst Pharm.* 1999 May 15;56(10):997–1000. Review.

19: Sanak M, Szczeklik A. Genetics of aspirin induced asthma. *Thorax.* 2000 Oct;55 Suppl 2:S45–7. Review.

20: Sprietsma JE. Modern diets and diseases: NO-zinc balance. Under Th1, zinc and nitrogen monoxide (NO) collectively protect against viruses, AIDS, autoimmunity, diabetes, allergies, asthma, infectious diseases, atherosclerosis and cancer. *Med Hypotheses.* 1999 Jul;53(1):6–16. Review.

21: Salinas AE, Wong MG. Glutathione S-transferases—a review. *Curr Med Chem.* 1999 Apr;6(4):279–309. Review.

22: von Mutius E. The burden of childhood asthma. *Arch Dis Child.* 2000 Jun;82 Suppl 2:II2–5. Review.

23: Fogarty A, Britton J. The role of diet in the aetiology of asthma. *Clin Exp Allergy.* 2000 May;30(5):615–27. Review.

24: Sicherer SH. Food allergy: when and how to perform oral food challenges. *Pediatr Allergy Immunol.* 1999 Nov;10(4):226–34. Review.

25: Williams C. Doing health, doing gender: teenagers, diabetes and asthma. *Soc Sci Med.* 2000 Feb;50(3):387–96. Review.

26: Cantani A, Gagliesi D. Prediction and prevention of allergic disease in at risk children. *Eur Rev Med Pharmacol Sci.* 1998 May–Aug;2(3-4):115–25. Review.

27: Sridhar MK. Nutrition and lung health. *Proc Nutr Soc.* 1999 May;58(2):303–8. Review.

CHAPTER 5

1: Warman KL. Management of asthma exacerbations: home treatment. *J Asthma.* 2000 Sep;37(6):461–8. Review.

2: Strachan DP. Family size, infection and atopy: the first decade of the "hygiene hypothesis". *Thorax.* 2000 Aug;55 Suppl 1:S2–10. Review.

3: Openshaw PJ, Hewitt C. Protective and harmful effects of viral infections in childhood on wheezing disorders and asthma. *Am J Respir Crit Care Med.* 2000 Aug;162(2 Pt 2):S40-3. Review.

4: Bush A, Tiddens H, Silverman M. Clinical implications of inflammation in young children. *Am J Respir Crit Care Med.* 2000 Aug;162(2 Pt 2):S11–4. Review.

5: Huang SW. Recent advances in the understanding of childhood asthma. *Taiwan Erh Ko I Hsueh Hui Tsa Chih.* 1999 May–Jun;40(3):145–51. Review.

6: Helms PJ. Corticosteroid-sparing options in the treatment of childhood asthma. *Drugs.* 2000;59 Suppl 1:15–22; discussion 43–5. Review.

7: Witzmann KBA, Fink RJ. Inhaled corticosteroids in childhood asthma: growing concerns. *Drugs.* 2000;59 Suppl 1:9–14; discussion 43–5. Review.

8: Nelson HS. Allergen and irritant control: importance and implementation. *Clin Cornerstone.* 1998 Aug–Sep;1(2):57–68. Review.

9: Miralles-Lopez J, Guillen-Grima F et al Bronchial asthma prevalence in childhood. *Allergol Immunopathol* (Madr). 1999 Jul–Aug;27(4):200–11. Review.

10: Clark NM, Brown RW et al. Childhood asthma. *Environ Health Perspect.* 1999 Jun;107 Suppl 3:421–9. Review.

11: Martinez FD. Maturation of immune responses at the beginning of asthma. *J Allergy Clin Immunol.* 1999 Mar;103(3 Pt 1):355-61. Review.

12: Boner AL, Bodini A, Piacentini GL. Environmental allergens and childhood asthma. *Clin Exp Allergy.* 1998 Nov;28 Suppl 5:76-81. Review.

CHAPTER 6

1. Bisgaard H. Role of leukotrienes in asthma pathophysiology. *Pediatr Pulmonol.* 2000 Aug;30(2):166–76. Review.

2: Holgate ST. The role of mast cells and basophils in inflammation. *Clin Exp Allergy.* 2000 Jun;30 Suppl 1:28–32. Review.

3: Paramesh H. Practical approach to recurrent respiratory infections. *Indian J Pediatr.* 1996 Mar-Apr;63(2):181–7. Review.

4: Amdekar YK, Ugra D. Pulmonary function tests. *Indian J Pediatr.* 1996 Mar–Apr;63(2):149–52. Review.

5: Clark CJ, Cochrane LM. Physical activity and asthma. *Curr Opin Pulm Med.* 1999 Jan;5(1):68–75. Review.

6: Ram FS, Robinson SM, Black PN. Physical training for asthma. *Cochrane Database Syst Rev.* 2000;(2):CD001116. Review.

7: DePalo VA, McCool FD. Exercise-induced asthma. *Med Health R I.* 2000 Feb;83(2):52–5. Review.

8: Packham S, Ebden P. Diagnosing and treating exercise-induced asthma. *Practitioner.* 1999 Nov;243(1604):830–1, 835–6. Review.

9: O'Byrne PM. Leukotriene bronchoconstriction induced by allergen and exercise. *Am J Respir Crit Care Med.* 2000 Feb;161(2 Pt 2):S68–72. Review.

10: Lowhagen O. Asthma and asthma-like disorders. *Respir Med.* 1999 Dec;93(12):851–5. Review.

11: Milgrom H, Taussig LM. Keeping children with exercise-induced asthma active. *Pediatrics.* 1999 Sep;104(3):e38. Review.

12: Inman MD. Management of exercise-induced bronchoconstriction. *Can Respir J.* 1999 Jul–Aug;6(4):345–54. Review.

13: Houtmeyers E, Gosselink R et al. Regulation of mucociliary clearance in health and disease. *Eur Respir J.* 1999 May;13(5):1177–88. Review.

14: Rietveld S, Everaerd W, Creer TL. Stress-induced asthma: a review of research and potential mechanisms. *Clin Exp Allergy.* 2000 Aug;30(8):1058–66. Review.

15: ten Thoren C, Petermann F. Reviewing asthma and anxiety. *Respir Med.* 2000 May;94(5):409–15. Review.

16: Bjorksten B. Unmet needs in the treatment of asthmatic children and adolescents: 2. *Clin Exp Allergy.* 2000 Jun;30 Suppl 1:73–6. Review.

17: Warner JO. Unmet needs in the treatment of asthmatic children and adolescents: 1. *Clin Exp Allergy.* 2000 Jun;30 Suppl 1:70–2. Review.

18: Juniper EF. Health-related quality of life in asthma. *Curr Opin Pulm Med.* 1999 Mar;5(2):105–10. Review.

19: Mellins RB, Evans D et al. Developing and communicating a long-term treatment plan for asthma. *Am Fam Physician.* 2000 Apr 15;61(8):2419–28, 2433–4. Review.

20: Sayer QM. Achieving compliance in asthma management. *Prof Nurse.* 1999 Nov;15(2):97–9. Review.

21: Bender BG, Annett RD. Neuropsychological outcomes of nocturnal asthma. *Chronobiol Int.* 1999 Sep;16(5):695–710. Review.

CHAPTER 7

1: Ziment I. Recent advances in alternative therapies. *Curr Opin Pulm Med.* 2000 Jan;6(1):71–8. Review.

2: Bielory L, Lupoli K. Herbal interventions in asthma and allergy. *J Asthma.* 1999;36(1):1–65. Review.

3: Birkel DA, Edgren L. Hatha yoga: improved vital capacity of college students. *Altern Ther Health Med.* 2000 Nov;6(6):55–63.

4: Krusche F. [Yoga respiratory therapy helps children with asthma]. *Fortschr Med.* 1999 Feb 20;117(5):44. .

5: Vedanthan PK, Kesavalu LN et al. Clinical study of yoga techniques in university students with asthma: a controlled study. *Allergy Asthma Proc.* 1998 Jan–Feb;19(1):3–9.

6: Lewith GT, Watkins AD. Unconventional therapies in asthma: an overview. *Allergy.* 1996 Nov;51(11):761–9. Review.

7: Bose S, Belapurkar N, Mishra U. Specific chiroglyphic, bronchial asthma and yoga. *J Assoc Physicians India.* 1992 Apr;40(4):279

8: Stanescu D. Yoga breathing exercises and bronchial asthma. *Lancet.* 1990 Nov 10;336(8724):1192.

9: Singh V, Wisniewski A, Britton J, Tattersfield A. Effect of yoga breathing exercises (pranayama) on airway reactivity in subjects with asthma. *Lancet.* 1990 Jun 9;335(8702):1381–3.

10: Singh V. Effect of respiratory exercises on asthma. The Pink City lung exercise. *J Asthma.* 1987;24(6):355–9.

CHAPTER 8

1: Byrd RP Jr, Krishnaswamy G, Roy TM. Difficult-to-manage asthma. How to pinpoint the exacerbating factors. *Postgrad Med.* 2000 Nov;108(6):37–40, 45–6, 49-50 passim.

2: Lippincott LL, Brown KR. Medical management of pediatric chronic sinusitis. *J La State Med Soc.* 2000 Oct;152(10):470–4.

3: Muller BA. Sinusitis and its relationship to asthma. Can treating one airway disease ameliorate another? *Postgrad Med.* 2000 Oct;108(5):55–61; quiz 13.

4: Lester MR, Schneider LC. Atopic diseases and upper respiratory infections. *Curr Opin Pediatr.* 2000 Oct;12(5):511–9.

5: Virant FS. Sinusitis and pediatric asthma. *Pediatr Ann.* 2000 Jul;29(7):434–7.

6: Altemeier WA 3rd, Graff GR. How are allergic rhinitis and sinusitis connected with asthma? *Pediatr Ann.* 2000 Jul;29(7):391–2, 398.

7: Walker SM, Pajno GB, Lima MT, Wilson DR, Durham SR. Grass pollen immunotherapy for seasonal rhinitis and asthma: A randomized, controlled trial. *J Allergy Clin Immunol.* 2001 Jan;107(1):87–93.

8: Droste JH, Wieringa MH et al. Does the use of antibiotics in early childhood increase the risk of asthma and allergic disease? *Clin Exp Allergy*. 2000 Nov;30(11):1548–53.

9: Seaton A, Devereux G. Diet, infection and wheezy illness: lessons from adults. *Pediatr Allergy Immunol*. 2000;11 Suppl 13:37–40.

10: Carvalho N, Fernandez-Benitez M et al. International study of asthma and allergies in childhood. Results on rhinitis of first phase in Pamplona, Spain. *Allergol Immunopathol* (Madr). 2000 Jul–Aug;28(4):207–12.

11: Plaschke PP, Janson C et al. Onset and remission of allergic rhinitis and asthma and the relationship with atopic sensitization and smoking. *Am J Respir Crit Care Med*. 2000 Sep;162(3 Pt 1):920–4.

12: Perez Martin J. [Comorbidity of rhinosinusitis and asthma]. *Rev Alerg Mex*. 2000 Jul–Aug;47(4):119–20.

13: Newson RB, Shaheen SO, Chinn S, Burney PG. Paracetamol sales and atopic disease in children and adults: an ecological analysis. *Eur Respir J*. 2000 Nov;16(5):817–23.

14: Behbehani NA, Abal A et al. Prevalence of asthma, allergic rhinitis, and eczema in 13- to 14-year-old children in Kuwait: an ISAAC study. International Study of Asthma and Allergies in Childhood. *Ann Allergy Asthma Immunol*. 2000 Jul;85(1):58–63.

15: Westerveld GJ, Dekker I, Voss HP, Bast A, Scheeren RA. Antioxidant levels in the nasal mucosa of patients with chronic sinusitis and healthy controls. *Arch Otolaryngol Head Neck Surg*. 1997 Feb;123(2):201–4.

16: Burch CR. Treatment of sinusitis and gingivitis. *Med J Aust*. 1977 May 28;1(22):831–2.

17: Lieu JE, Feinstein AR. Confirmations and surprises in the association of tobacco use with sinusitis. *Arch Otolaryngol Head Neck Surg*. 2000 Aug;126(8):940–6.

CHAPTER 9

1: Taylor JP, Krondl MM, Csima AC. Assessing adherence to a rotary diversified diet, a treatment for 'environmental illness'. *J Am Diet Assoc*. 1998 Dec;98(12):1439–44.

2: Krop JJ. Treatment and prophylaxis for patients suffering from environmental hypersensitivity disorder. *Folia Med Cracov*. 1993;34(1–4):159–72.

3: [No authors listed]. Clinical ecology. American College of Physicians. *Ann Intern Med*. 1989 Jul 15;111(2):168–78. Review.

4: Bahna SL. Management of food allergies. *Ann Allergy*. 1984 Dec;53(6 Pt 2):678–82. Review.

5: Hall K. Allergy of the nervous system: a review. *Ann Allergy*. 1976 Jan;36(1):49–64. Review.

CHAPTER **12**

1. Aao K. The biochemistry of food allergens: What is essential for future research? *In Food Allergy* Reinhardt D and Schmidt E . Eds. 1988:Raven Press, New York.

2. Ames BN et al. Dietary pesticides (99.9% all natural) *Proc. Natl. Acad. Sci. USA* (1990) 87:7777 & 87: 7782.

3. Brusse W. Viruses in Asthma. *J Aller Clin Immunol.* 1997; 100(2):147-50.

4. Bykowski. Allergies can touch off asthma attacks. *Skin and Allergy News* July (1997); 21.

5. Davidson AG et al. Coeliac disease: an analysis of aetiological possibilities and re-evaluation of the enzymopathic hypothesis. *Med Hypotheses.* 1988;26(3):155-160.

6. Gardner RW. Chemical intolerance: Physiological causes and effects and treatment modalities. 1994:CRC Press Inc.

7. Korkmaz ME et al. Levels of IgE in the Serum of Patients with Coronary Arterial Disease. *Int J. Cardiol.* 1991;31(2):199-204.

8. Isolauni E. Intestinal involvement in Atopic disease. *J. Royal Society of Med.* 1997:90 (suppl 30) 15:20

9. Jeffrey GT. A critical analysis of multiple chemical sensititivities. *Med Hypotheses.* 1998;50:303-311.

10. Mounir Fouad F Marshall WD.& Farrell PG. On the Genesis of Gastric Haemorrhage. *Med Hypotheses* 1989;30:131-134.

11. Plant et al. New directions in food allergy research. *J Aller Clin Immunol.* 1997;100 (1) 7-10.

12. Rodriguez J et al. Occupational asthma caused by fish inhalation. *Allergy.* 1997;52:866-869

13. Schuppan D et al. Exposing gliadin as a tasty food for lymphocytes. *Nature Med.* 1998;4(6):666-7.

14. Wutrich B. Oral Allergy Syndrome. *Allergy Network.* 1997;27633.

15. Alessandro F. Exercise-Induced Anaphylaxis After Food Contaminant Ingestion in a Double-Blinded, Placebo-Controlled, Food-Exercise Challenge. *Journal of Allergy and Clinical Immunology,* September, 1997;100(3):424-425.

16. Broughton KS et al. Reduced asthma symptoms with n-3 fatty acid ingestion are related to 5-series leukotriene production. *Am J Clin Nutr.* 1997;65(4):1011-1017.

17. Cohen HA. Blocking effect of vitamin C in exercise-induced asthma. *Arch Pediatr Adolesc Med.* 1997;151(4):367-370.

18. Dinh Xuan AT. Bronchial Blood Flow and Microvascular Permeability in the Pathophysiology of Asthma. *Med Hypotheses.* 1990;32(3):207-209

19. Garin PR & Frans A. Aspirin - Relieved Asthma. *Med Hypotheses.* 1990;32(20:125-128.

20. Hauser SP et al. Intravenous magnesium administration in bronchial asthma. *Schweiz Med Wochenschr* 1989;199(46):1633-1635.

21. Hillel S. Asthma and the Environment. *Environmental Health Perspectives*, 1997;105(5):533-537.

22. Holst PE. Management of Asthma in Pregnancy .*Current Therapeutics* March 1985: 61-66.

23. Kashalikar SJ. A Common Denominator in the Pathogenesis of Asthma. *Med Hypotheses*. 1988;27(4):255-259.

24. Nguyen Myngoc T. Effect of Cow Milk on Pulmonary Function in Atopic Asthmatic Patients. *Annals of Allergy, Asthma and Immunology*, 1997;79(1):62-64. 28108

25. Phelan PD. Symptomatic Treatment of Cough in Children Current Therapeutics April 1986, 77-81

26. Plaut M. New Directions in Food Allergy Research,. *Journal of Allergy and Clinical Immunology* July, 1997;100(1):7-10.

27. Reynolds RD et al. Depressed plasma pyridoxal phosphate concentrations in adult asthmatics *Am J Clin Nutr*. 1985;41(4);684-688.

28. Rosival V. The role of pulmonary hypertension in the pathogenesis of bronchial asthma. *Med Hypotheses* 1990;33(1):7-9.

29. Sibbald B. Extrinsic and Intrinsic Asthma: influence of Classification on Family History of Asthma and Allergic Disease. *Clin Allergy*, 1980;10: 313-318

30. Soutar A. Bronchial reactivity and dietary antioxidants. *Thorax* 1997;52(2):166-170.

31. Tanaka I et al. Serum concentrrations of the pyridoxal and pyridoxal -5-phosphate in children during sustained-release theophylline therapy. *Arerugi* 1996;45(10):1098-1105.

32. Weiss ST. Diet as a risk factor for asthma. *Ciba Found Symp* 1997;206: 44-257.

33. Gassner-Bachmann M et al. Farmers'children suffer less from hayfever and asthma. *Dtsch Med Wochenschr*. 2000 Aug 4;125(31-32):924-31.

34. Marshall GD et al. Stess, immuneregulation, and immunity: applications for asthma. *Allergy Asthma Proc*. 2000 Jul-Aug;21(4):241-6.

35. Sprietsma JE. Modern diets and diseases: NO-zinc balance. Under Th1, zinc and nitrogen monoxide (NO) collectively protect against viruses, AIDS, autoimmunity, diabetes, allergies, asthma, infectious diseases, atherosclerosis and cancer. *Med Hypotheses* 1999 Jul;53(1):6-16. Review.

36. Huss K et al. House dust mite and cockroach exposure are strong risk factors for positive allergy skin test responses in the Childhood Asthma Management Program. *J Allergy Clin Immunol*. 2001 Jan;107(1):48-54

37. Foucard T. Is prevention of allergy and asthma possible. *Acta Paediatr Suppl.* 200 Sep;89(434 suppl):71-5.

38. Naakura T et al. Dietary supplementation of fish oil rich in omega-3 polyunsaturated fatty acids in children with bronchial asthma. *Eur Respir J.* 2000 Nov;16(5):861-5.

39. Okamato M et al. Effects of dietary supplementation with n-3 fatty acids compared with n-6 fatty acid on bronchial asthma. *Intern Med.* 2000 Feb;39(2):107-11.

40. Schwartz J. Role of polyunsaturated fatty acids in lung disease. *Am J Clin Nutr.* 2000 Jan;71(1 Suppl):393S-6S. Review.

41. Heller A et al. Lipid mediators in inflammatory disorders. *Drugs* 1998 Apr;55(4):487-96. Review.

42. Shimizu T et al . Relation between theophylline and circulating vitamin levels in children with asthma. *Pharmacology.* 1996 Dec;53(6):384-9.

43. Bielory L et al. Asthma and vitamin C. *Ann Allergy.* 1994 Aug;73(2):89-96 Review.

44. Fogarty A et al. The role of diet in the aetiology of asthma. *Clin Exp Allergy.* 200 May;30(5):615-27 Review.

45. Saris NF et al. Magnesium. An update on physiological, clinical and analytical aspects. *Clin Chim Acta* 2000 Apr;294(1-2):1-26 Review.

46. Sicherer SH. Food Allergy: when and how to perform oral food challenges. *Pediatr Allergy Immunol.* 199 Nov;10(4):226-34 Review.

47. Vural H et al. Serum and red blood cell antioxidant status in patients with bronchial asthma. *Can Respir J.* 2000 Nov;7(6):476-480.

48. Fogarty A et al. Dietary E, IgE concentrations, and atopy. *Lancet* 2000 Nov4;356(9241):1573-4.

49. Baker JC et al Dietary antioxidants and magnesium in type 1 brittle asthma: a case control study. *Thorax.* 1999 Feb;54(2):115-8

50. Soutar A et al. Bronchial reactivity and dietary antioxidants. *Thorax* 1997 Feb;52(2):166-70.

51. Platts-Mills TA et al. Changing concepts of allergic disease: the attempt to keep up with real changes in lifestyles. *J Allergy Clin Immunol* 1996 Dec;98(6 Pt 3):S297-306. Review.

52. William J. Rea Chemical sensitivity Volume 2; Source of total body load . Lewis Publishers 1994.

53. Robert W. Gardner. *Chemical Intolerance: Physiological Causes and Effects and Treatment Modalities.* CRC Press 1994.

INDEX

149

Henry Osiecki graduated from the University of Queensland, Australia with an Honors Degree in Science, majoring in physiology and pharmacology. He received his Post Graduate Diploma in Nutrition and Dietetics from Queensland Institute of Technology. Mr. Osiecki has authored papers in kidney research, cancer, sports nutrition, and Down's Syndrome and has published a textbook in clinical nutrition that is used in naturopathic colleges throughout Australia. An international lecturer in clinical nutrition at universities, colleges and professional seminars, Henry has also produced several popular radio programs on health and nutrition.

Mr. Osiecki has practiced as a consulting nutritionist/dietitian for the past twenty years. His success has led to an overwhelming public demand for his services as well as an increasing amount of press, radio and television coverage. A true pioneer in the field of health, Mr. Osiecki has made an enormous contribution to the health and well-being of thousands of people. His other books include:

Hypernutrition for Sport,
Nutrients in Profile,
and
The Physician's Handbook
of Clinical Nutrition.

OTHER TITLES FROM
VITAL HEALTH PUBLISHING:

Stevia Sweet Recipes: Sugar-Free - Naturally! (2nd ed.), Jeffrey Goettemoeller, 200 pages, 1-890612-13-8, $13.95.

Stevia Rebaudiana: Nature's Sweet Secret (3rd ed.), David Richard, includes stevia growing information, 80 pages, 1-890612-15-4, $7.95.

Nutrition in a Nutshell: Build Health and Slow Down the Aging Process, Bonnie Minsky, L.C.N., M.A.,. approx 160 pages, 1-890612-17-0, $12.95.

Wheatgrass: Superfood for a New Millenium, Li Smith, 164 pages, 1-890612-10-3, $10.95.

Energy For Life: How to Overcome Chronic Fatigue, George Redmon, Ph.D., N.D. approx. 240 pages, 1-890612-14-6, $15.95.

The Cancer Handbook: What's Really Working, edited by Lynne McTaggart, 192 pages, 1-890612-18-9, $12.95.

Taste Life! The Organic Choice, Ed. by David Richard and Dorie Byers, R.N., 208 pages, 1-890612-08-1, $12.95.

Lecithin and Health, Frank Orthoefer, Ph.D., 80 pages, 1-890612-03-0, $8.95.

Natural Beauty Basics: Making Your Own Cosmetics and Body Care Products, Dorie Byers, R.N., 208 pages, 1-890612-19-7, $14.95.

Anoint Yourself With Oil for Radiant Health, David Richard, 56 pages, 1-890612-01-4, $7.95.

My Whole Food ABC's, David Richard and Susan Cavaciuti, 28 color pages, children's, 1-890612-07-3, $8.95

Healing Herb Rapid Reference, Brent Davis, D.C., 148 pages, 1-890612-21-9, $12.95.

OTHER TITLES
FROM ENHANCEMENT BOOKS:

The Veneration of Life: Through the Disease to the Soul, John Diamond, M.D., 80 pages, 1-890995-14-2, $9.95.

The Way of the Pulse: Drumming With Spirit, John Diamond, M.D., 116 pages, 1-890995-02-9, $13.95.

The Healing Power of Blake: A Distillation, edited by John Diamond, M.D., 180 pages, 1-890995-03-7, $14.95.

The Healer: Heart and Hearth, John Diamond, M.D., 112 pages, 1-890995-22-3, $13.95.

Life Enhancement Through Music, John Diamond, M.D., approx. 176 pages, 1-890995-01-0, $14.95.

Facets of a Diamond: Aspects of a Healer, John Diamond, M.D., approx. 400 pages, 1-890995-17-7, $22.95.

Someone Hurt Me, Susan Cavaciuti, 48 pages, color illustrated, children's, 1-890995-20-7, $8.95.

Vital Health Publishing/Enhancement Books
P.O. Box 544
Bloomingdale, IL 60108
(630) 876-0426
Website: www.vitalhealth.net
Email: vitalhealth@compuserve.com